LET'S TALK ABOUT SLEEP

LET'S TALK ABOUT SLEEP

A Guide to Understanding and Improving Your Slumber

Daniel A. Barone, MD, with Lawrence A. Armour

ROWMAN & LITTLEFIELD
Lanham • Boulder • New York • London

Published by Rowman & Littlefield
A wholly owned subsidiary of The Rowman & Littlefield Publishing Group, Inc.
4501 Forbes Boulevard, Suite 200, Lanham, Maryland 20706
www.rowman.com

Unit A, Whitacre Mews, 26-34 Stannary Street, London SE11 4AB

British Library Cataloguing in Publication Information Available

Library of Congress Cataloging-in-Publication Data Is Available

ISBN 978-1-5381-0398-2 (cloth: alk. paper)
ISBN 978-1-5381-0399-9 (electronic)

♾ ™ The paper used in this publication meets the minimum requirements of American National Standard for Information Sciences Permanence of Paper for Printed Library Materials, ANSI/NISO Z39.48-1992.

Printed in the United States of America

CONTENTS

INTRODUCTION

Hamlet in his famous "To be or not to be" soliloquy refers to sleep, specifically "to sleep, perchance to dream," but Shakespeare was hardly the first to weigh in on the subject and delve into how sleep impacts our brain, mind, body, and soul.

In fact, writers of the Bible, the Ancient Egyptians, Socrates, Plato, and Aristotle, to name a few, had fascinating things to say about sleep. And what is even more interesting is that much of what the early societies thought about proper sleep is actually relevant today, with all that we now know about sleep and sleep disorders.

In Ancient Greece, for example, sleep and death were considered close relatives. In Homer's famous work *The Iliad*, the gods Hypnos and Thanatos, twin brothers, were described as Hypnos being the god of sleep and Thanatos the god of death. Through the descriptions of these gods, we can see what the Ancient Greeks thought about sleep (and death, for that matter: Thanatos's sword was symbolic of the belief that the soul was separated from the body at time of death). Hypnos was often depicted reclining in fields of poppies (known to induce sleep), and in settings with the Greek gods of medicine, and he was considered to be a consoler of souls. We now know the impact healthy sleep has on both body and mind, and given the ancient Greek view of it through descriptions of Hypnos, it is clear they were aware of this as well.[1]

Another example of the many ways past societies had real wisdom regarding sleep can be found in the Islamic tradition. The prophet

Muhammad outlined the right way for his followers to live, which included advice on how to sleep. He advised them to "lie on [their] right side," among other recommendations.[2] We have no idea if Muhammad or any of his followers actually suffered from the condition known as obstructive sleep apnea, but it turns out his suggestion is a good way to deal with it. As we will learn in detail later on, obstructive sleep apnea is a common disorder in which there are repeated stoppages of breathing while someone is asleep. Usually the stoppages of breathing occur because the tongue and/or soft tissues fall toward the back of the throat. Sleeping on the side not only may reduce or eliminate obstructive sleep apnea, but it is also the most neutral position for one's neck (with head supported on a pillow) and spine.

We have all heard of, and probably experienced, insomnia at some point in our lives. It is defined as difficulty falling asleep, difficulty staying asleep, and/or sleep that is not restorative. As we will get into later, one of the ways to improve sleep, and potentially treat insomnia, is with proper sleep hygiene. Sleep hygiene is a collection of practices that aid in healthy sleep when done correctly. Part of good sleep hygiene is sticking to a routine daily sleep-and-wake schedule. In the Old Testament (Psalm 57:9; 108:3), the proper timing of sleep is alluded to: "Awake, O, my soul. Awake, O harp and lyre! I will wake the dawn." This passage implies that the sleep period should end at the same time each day, and that one should not sleep in.[3] Similarly, a recommendation is made in the Talmud[4] about making one's bed environment dark. A cool, dark bedroom is another aspect of good sleep hygiene and can be an effective countermeasure against insomnia.

Finally, the Ancient Chinese utilized the pulse as an important tool in the diagnosis of disease. First mentioned in the classic work of internal medicine *Nei Ching*, written by the Yellow Emperor, Huang Ti (698–598 BCE), the pulse was thought to reflect the interaction between yin (disease) and yang (health).[5] The ancient Chinese physicians judged the state of disease by the volume, strength, weakness, regularity, or interruption of a patient's pulse.[6] Today, researchers are looking into heart-rate variability (which is one aspect of some of the research that I do[7]) as one measure of a person's health—this is fascinating to me because it coincides with the ancient Chinese traditional understanding of the heart, which they noted was the "seat of consciousness," and played a major role in insomnia. We know today that those with chronic insomnia are at greater risk for heart-related problems, and one small piece of evidence for this is seen with measurements of heart-rate variability.[8]

These early insights into sleep health are fascinating to talk and think about, and I mentioned just a few of the many that have been reported. But what is definitely shown to us through them is that our current age is not the first to think about and opine on the various aspects of sleep. To this point, nowadays, news about sleep is everywhere we turn, accompanied by an avalanche of numbing statistics. In case you missed them, here are a few:

- According to the National Institutes of Health, fifty to seventy million Americans are affected by chronic sleep disorders and intermittent sleep problems.[9]
- Some 30–35 percent of adults complain of insomnia.[10]
- One in every twenty-five Americans takes a prescription sleep medication.[11]
- More than a third of American adults are not getting enough sleep on a regular basis.[12]
- Sleep disorders account for an estimated $16 billion in medical costs each year, plus indirect costs due to missed days of work, decreased productivity, and related factors.[13]

But forget the statistics for a second. What happens to the brain when we sleep is one of the most fascinating and mysterious questions in all of science. Questions such as: "What is the environment on other planets like?" "What is a star composed of?" and "Do other galaxies exist?" have all been answered—but why do we sleep? What happens when we sleep? We know biochemically what is happening in the brain, and that in sleep the brain is still active, but what about the mind? What about the soul? And what about dreams? We believe that an aspect of consciousness is preserved in dreams, but what does that tell us about consciousness?

I've been fascinated by sleep for years. Through this book, my goal is to share—in a friendly, readable way—the highlights of what I have learned and what I share with my patients on a daily basis. We will discuss—in terms everyone can understand—what we know about sleep, what can go wrong with it, and what we can do to fix it. To add a fresh dimension, we have included firsthand stories of people who suffer from sleep disorders and what they have done to deal with them.

Along the way on our sleep journey, we will take a look at the conditions you may have heard or read about, such as obstructive sleep apnea and insomnia, mentioned above. But we also will be delving into sleep problems you may not have even known existed—things like narcolepsy, exploding head syndrome, restless legs syndrome, and sexsomnia.

Additionally, we will be talking about the popular medications out there to treat sleep; we will go into what they are, how they work, and if they are effective. As you will soon see, I prefer to try natural remedies first with my patients, if the situation permits. For example, you are going to read about the natural supplement known as melatonin, a hormone made by our brains daily that can now be taken in pill form. And about the sleep-inducing properties of a plant known as valerian.

I'm certain you are constantly inundated with advertisements of new technologies and apps that are popping up on an almost daily basis. We will discuss these and look at whether or not they are truly effective in promoting sleep.

We will close the book with a discussion of dreams—what they may mean, what research has shown us about them, and what the brilliant minds of both science and spirituality have said about them.

While you can read this book cover to cover, and I hope you do, don't see it as an assignment. Feel free to skip around or jump to a chapter that pertains to a problem you or a loved one may be suffering from.

I had fun writing this book. In addition to finding useful information and suggestions that will improve all aspects of your life, I hope you have fun reading it.

—Daniel A. Barone, MD, 2017

I

TROUBLE SLEEPING?

You're not the only one. Fortunately, there are steps you can take to help yourself.

Sleep disorders come in many forms: insomnia, sleep apnea, other things you've undoubtedly heard about, and others that may be new to you. Sometimes trouble stems from the fact we've become a twenty-four-hour society. We work when we get home at night. We're constantly on the Internet. We're constantly on the phone. We think about problems when we get into bed. We do everything but sleep.

As a society, we sleep one hour less per night than our ancestors did, and while that may not sound like much, it actually is very significant. I'll explain. The average adult needs seven to nine hours of sleep each night,[1] and when deprived, the short-term consequences can be just what you'd think: poor concentration, irritability, and daytime sleepiness and/or fatigue. Now, let's suppose a person only gets six hours per night through the week (when they really need eight). After a week of this, the sleep "debt" adds up to the equivalent of one night without sleep. And that, as you might imagine, can have a deleterious effect not only on one's concentration and mood, but also on one's health over time.

Lack of sleep can cause blood pressure to go up and increase the risk of cardiovascular illness later in life. It can have other ill effects, including, as was confirmed in a study from 2016, increasing the risk of catching a cold.[2] There's also an association between how sleep deprived we are and our cognitive performance. People who are sleep deprived are at an increased risk for car accidents. In fact, the day after daylight savings is the number one day for car accidents in America.[3] That's because we are sleep deprived to begin with, and pushing the clock ahead takes another hour out of our sleep time.

So what can we do about it? We will be talking about many of the causes that reduce sleep quality and/or quantity throughout this book, as well as the treatments for them. To start off, however, I thought it would be a good idea to relay some sleep hygiene tips. Sleep hygiene, as you may recall from the introduction, is a strange term that we use to describe a collection of practices that aid in healthy sleep. You can think of them as sleep guidelines. Proper sleep hygiene is not *direly* needed in those without sleep problems, but I do recommend everyone trying to incorporate them into their daily/nightly routine to prevent such issues in the future. And as for those suffering with insomnia or other chronic sleep disorders, good sleep hygiene is a must:

- Avoid caffeine, alcohol, nicotine, and other chemicals that interfere with sleep. Ideally, these all should be eliminated. If you want a drink, maybe a glass of wine with dinner would be okay. And what I tell my patients if they have trouble sleeping, no caffeine or even decaf coffee after 1 p.m. Same thing with nicotine; if you're not able to eliminate it completely, as least limit it to the daytime.
- Turn your bedroom into a sleep-inducing environment. You want the bedroom to be a little on the cool side and as dark as you can make it. I recommend blackout shades. When the sun starts coming up, the little bit of light that creeps in can wake you or, if you're already up, it can make it very hard to get back to sleep.
- The TV, tablet, computer, smartphone, and all aspects of the work environment should be out of your bedroom. Thirty to sixty minutes before you plan to get into bed, shut off all "blue light" devices—that includes all of the above. The blue light refers to the type of light that these devices produce. Blue light sends a message to our brain to shut off its production of melatonin. As we will see later, melatonin production begins the process of allowing us to sleep.
- Regarding the blue light issue, some companies have incorporated blue light "blocking" technology into their devices. These de-

vices are able to produce screen images without use of blue light (by using other colors). While the science behind it makes sense, I always tell my patients to just stop with the devices altogether, as I mentioned above. A quick rule of thumb is that if the screen can be seen without an external light (in other words, if it is back lit), it's better to shut it off thirty to sixty minutes prior to bedtime.

• Establish a soothing pre-sleep routine. For example, utilizing meditation (see the section following this list), listening to soft music, and taking a warm bath or stretching before bed can all be effective. Or, do as Mom says, and give a glass of warm milk a try.

• Go to bed when you're truly tired. Sometimes, patients with insomnia will get into bed early in an attempt to try to get extra sleep. This unfortunately rarely works, and you're actually better off delaying your bedtime until you're really tired.

• Don't be a clock watcher. This is a big thing. Patients who have insomnia often lie there, continuously looking at the clock, counting down the minutes, getting frustrated. If you want to set an alarm, that's fine, but turn it away from you or put it facedown. You don't want the temptation of checking the clock to see what time it is, as doing so may make you more anxious and not be of any help.

• Use light to your advantage. When you wake up in the morning, particularly if you have trouble sleeping, getting twenty minutes or so of sunlight can really help; ideally this should be done outside and as close to wake time as possible. Then, when you go to sleep, sleep in a dark environment.

• Keep your internal clock set with a consistent sleep schedule. I find one common problem is with weekends, when people go to bed a little later and then sleep in. If you go to bed late Saturday, then sleep in on Sunday, you might have difficulty getting to sleep on Sunday night, which then can throw your entire sleep schedule off. You want to be as consistent as possible, maybe within an hour or so, with your sleep and wake-up times. They should be the same on weekdays as on weekends.

• Start a "worry" journal that you use at least a few hours before your planned bedtime. If you have things on your mind, write them down in two columns. List the problems or things you're worrying about in the left column, and write the solutions in the right column. Say, for example, tomorrow you've got a meeting with your boss. In the right column, list the things you did to prepare for the meeting. You did all the things you needed to do, so you don't have to worry about that. There seems to be some benefit getting it out into the open, leaving less chance you'll take it with you to bed. Keep a paper and pen next to your bed so if you wake from sleep worrying or thinking about something, you can write it down and address it in the morning.

- Nap early or not at all. If you absolutely need a nap, it should be only fifteen to twenty minutes, maybe thirty minutes in length, and as early in the day as possible. After getting home from work, eating dinner, and watching the evening news, some people doze off and sleep for fifteen minutes. This is technically a nap. As we stay awake throughout the day, our brain gets tired and sleep pressure builds up, which is our drive to fall asleep. When we take a nap in the evening, we may reduce our sleep pressure for the night, making it difficult to fall asleep. By avoiding that, you help your body fall asleep at nighttime.
- Lighten up on evening meals. You do not want to go to bed with a full stomach, but you also don't want to go to bed hungry. If it's close to bedtime and you're hungry, try a small snack, maybe like a few nuts, something to fill your stomach but nothing too heavy.
- Cut back on fluids toward the end of the day. You want to drink eight glasses of water a day, but it's good to cut back as the evening goes along. Try not to drink anything an hour or two before bed because that can trigger an awakening.
- Exercise regularly. It has been shown that regular cardiovascular exercise can help with sleep,[4] but try to do it at least a few hours before you are planning to go to bed. Early in the morning is best.
- You should think of the bedroom as your temple of sleep, and anything that can "desecrate" this temple should be removed. Essentially, the bed and even the bedroom should only be used for sleeping or for being intimate. Anything else may confuse the brain as to what the bed environment is really for and can make sleeping problems harder to fix.
- Avoid snoozing. The process of waking up is not like an on-off switch; it is based on neurochemicals being released at the right times. Therefore, when we snooze and head back to sleep (which

does feel good, I agree) we are reversing this process abruptly. Waking up once again will then throw off the brain's chemistry, and you may feel worse or "out of it" for a few hours. It is better to just set your alarm for the latest time you can wake up, and then just get up at that time.

- Last but far from least, follow through on all the above. These improvements do not work immediately. It may take a couple of weeks for the body to adjust to them. So it's necessary to follow through with all the recommendations as best you can.

To shift gears slightly, I would like to end this chapter with a simple introduction to *mindfulness meditation*, which is one of the most powerful techniques out there for relaxing and calming the mind. With this form of meditation you are *paying mind* to breathing, which can help clear your head, which may, in turn, help you get to sleep a little easier.

There are many different resources to turn to for instructions on meditation and many different videos you can look at. (Simply type "mindfulness meditation" or "how to meditate" into a search engine and you'll get thousands of good YouTube results.) But let me walk you through the way I tell my patients how to meditate.

Start by finding a quiet environment. Sit at the edge of the bed or up in a chair in an area that's nice and relaxing to you. Turn off the lights and have soft music playing if you like, or just do it in silence.

Close your eyes, get into a relaxed position with your hands on your lap, and keep your eyes closed. Breathe in through your nose and out through your mouth in a nice, slow, controlled way. *In through the nose, out through the mouth.* And as you're doing this, focus on your breathing. If it helps, imagine images of air moving into your nose and out through your mouth. Or say "in" as you breathe in and "out" as you breathe out. Do whatever helps you concentrate on your breathing.

As you're doing this, you're probably going to have thoughts about what happened during the day or what is happening in your life. Don't try to block those thoughts out; just acknowledge them and then bring your attention back to your breathing. That's your home base. *In through the nose, out through the mouth.*

After you do this for a few minutes, I want you to begin to feel the muscles in your body start to relax. Starting with the neck and shoulders, feel those muscles become less tense. As you continue to focus on breathing in through the nose and out through the mouth, notice the sense of relaxation move down to your chest muscles, then to your abdominal muscles, and then down to your upper legs and lower legs, to your feet, and even the tips of your toes. Let everything progressively relax as you concentrate on breathing. *In through the nose and out through the mouth.*

Do this during the day if you like—any time you feel stressed you can do a quick session—but certainly do it fifteen to thirty minutes or so before bedtime. Make meditation part of your ritual. Instead of watching TV or working on your computer, make it a point to practice mindfulness meditation for ten to fifteen minutes each night. This technique can also be used in the middle of the night to help you get back to sleep, and I often recommend it just for this circumstance. If meditation becomes part of your daily routine, it can help make your mind clear and your body more relaxed, and it may improve your sleep.

SUMMARY

The key things to remember from this chapter are as follows:

- Sleep problems are very common. If you or a family member suffers from one, you are not alone.
- Good sleep habits are essential for healthy sleep. Work hard to turn your sleep time into a priority (without putting unnecessary pressure on yourself) and your sleep environment into a "temple" of sorts.
- Mindfulness meditation can be a very effective aid in getting to sleep or getting back to sleep. You should really consider using this as a completely natural and safe resource.

2

THE BRAIN

What Happens When We Sleep?

The brain is essentially a sponge-like mass a little bigger than a fist. It's wrinkly, slippery, and looks kind of whitish gray. Within this mass of tissue lies the basis for everything we think and do.

If we take a microscope and move in very close, we see that the brain is composed of nerve cells called neurons. These neurons talk to each other through electrical signals, and that "conversation" is what produces everything we regard as being conscious and alive.

Groups of neurons within the brain join together to form bigger and bigger structures. We ultimately end up with lobes of the brain (the frontal, parietal, temporal, and occipital) and other structures such as the suprachiasmatic nucleus and the pineal gland, which we will discuss in a minute. These lobes and structures have particular functions. All are subject to the effects of sleep, and all play a role in initiating or maintaining sleep.

So "how" do we sleep? The process of falling asleep and waking up is not like an on-and-off switch. In the natural state (i.e., in the wilderness without electronics or artificial light), the process of falling asleep typically begins once it gets dark outside. As this happens, special cells in our eyes send a signal to an area of our brain called the suprachiasmatic nucleus (SCN). The SCN gets its name because it sits above the optic chasm, which is where signals from the eye cross to the opposite side of the brain. Once the SCN gets word that it is getting dark outside, it sends a signal to the pineal gland, which produces melatonin; melatonin, which we'll discuss later, is one of the main hormones of the brain, and once it is released, the process that ultimately results in sleep begins.

Conversely, sunlight and a form of artificial light that comes from screens (tablets, smartphones, TVs, computers, etc.), known as "blue light," tell the brain to shut off the production of melatonin. By shutting off melatonin, the signal to *not* sleep is triggered. I know this sounds confusing, but the bottom line to remember is that light plays a major role in when we sleep, and the pineal gland is a big part of this process.

Throughout history, when people dissected humans in an effort to figure out why and how we sleep, the pineal gland was one of the prominent structures examined. Its name comes from the fact that it looks like a pinecone. It sits in the actual center of the brain and is one of the only unpaired structures in the brain. For these reasons, it was always considered to have special properties.

In Aristotle and Plato's time, people thought the pineal gland acted as a valve that allowed vapors to rise from the feet to the brain, and that was the process that caused us to fall asleep. Rene Descartes, the famous Renaissance philosopher who is known for "I think, therefore I am," believed the pineal gland to be where the soul resides. Others, including members of various Hindu traditions, viewed the pineal gland as a "third eye" that provides access to the unseen spirit world. Even today, there are many fascinating theories on the metaphysical properties of the pineal gland (including some interesting ones that are rooted in conspiracy theories). The one thing we know for sure is what it does biologically: it produces melatonin.

What has always fascinated me is how the process of going from a "wake state" to a "sleep state" occurs. Think about it: we never remember the exact moment at which sleep onset occurs, so at what point have enough of the nerve cells "crossed over"? It is an interesting question to ponder, one that was brought to my attention after reading *The Stanford Sleep Book*, which was written by the father of sleep medicine, Dr. William Dement. No one really knows, but like many things in science and medicine, with time it may be discovered.

What we do know from personal experiences and hard science is that we absolutely need sleep. The big question is: "How much?" The "average" person needs seven to nine hours of sleep per night. Many people are not getting that.[1]

This is not to say that everyone requires the same amount of sleep. Some people are short sleepers who get by on four or five hours a night. For these people, it's possible that their brains are just more "efficient." In other words, they get a higher percentage of the deeper forms of sleep in a short period of time compared to people who need eight hours of sleep.

As an interesting offshoot of this idea, there are scientific studies of Buddhist monks and others who meditate intensively. The studies, utilizing a special type of imaging known as functional MRI, have found that after months and months of hard-core meditation, the amount of sleep a person needs can drop substantially because, as the theory goes, the brain becomes more efficient.[2]

Conversely, some adults need nine to ten hours (or more) of sleep per night. We call them long sleepers. As an aside, I would not categorize someone as a "long sleeper" without first making sure there was not another sleep issue present. For example, because the quality of their sleep is impaired, people with sleep apnea may actually need more sleep per night if they are left untreated.

So, what exactly is happening when we sleep? Contrary to popular belief, when we fall asleep, our brain doesn't simply shut off. In many cases, our brain is just as active as it was when awake. Furthering this point, the brain cycles through various stages of sleep through the night.[3] We know this from many studies examining brain waves of people (technically known as an electroencephalogram, EEG) during wakefulness and sleep.[4]

Most people have heard of REM sleep, which is rapid eye movement sleep, so named because our eyes literally move in a rapid fashion back and forth during this stage of sleep.[5] While our eyes are darting rapidly side to side, our body is *completely* paralyzed (except, of course, our main breathing muscle, called the diaphragm, and a small muscle in our ears). You can see if someone is in REM sleep by watching the person's eyes under the eyelids: if there seems to be rapid darting back and forth, there is a good chance it is REM sleep. We actually dream through the night, but our dreams tend to be most active in REM sleep. By paralyzing our bodies, nature has decided that we should not be acting out those dreams.

Through the night, REM sleep is intermixed with the creatively named non-REM (NREM) sleep, which ranges from light to deep. We transition from stage to stage in approximately ninety-minute cycles as the night goes along, and each cycle ends with a period of REM sleep. We then may wake up and fall right back asleep, or the cycle may repeat without an awakening.

When we look at a person's brain during quiet wakefulness with eyes closed, the brain waves (EEG) are close together—we call these "alpha waves." As we enter into light sleep, our brain waves spread apart a little bit—we call this NREM stage 1, or simply N1. We spend about 5–15 percent of our night in this very light form of sleep, which is very easy to wake up from. Imagine falling asleep on a subway or train for ten minutes on the way home from work; there is a good chance you would be in N1 sleep.

As our sleep gets deeper and deeper, the brain waves get more spread out, and we end up spending the majority of the night in this stage of sleep known as N2. About 45–55 percent of our night is spent in N2, and we think of it as the "baseline" of sleep. In this stage, there are odd-looking waves called K complexes and sleep spindles.

Eventually, the brain waves get bigger and more spread apart, which is when we achieve N3 sleep, also referred to as "delta wave" or "slow wave" sleep. This very deep sleep is extremely difficult to wake up from, and tends to occur in the first half of the night. Children tend to have much more of this type of sleep, probably to help their brains as they are maturing. We spend about 20–25 percent of our night here.

We move through these different stages of NREM sleep and end with a period of REM, a cycle that happens four to five times per night. We spend about 20–25 percent of the night in REM, and the REM periods get longer and longer as the night goes along, which is why we sometimes wake up out of a dream.

This is a good point to pause and take a look at the differences in the two "important" stages of sleep. I used quotations because all sleep is important, but REM and N3 are the ones usually impacted by sleep disorders. We talked about REM sleep and how it is essentially dream sleep; some researchers believe that REM dream sleep helps us form and store memories and improve our overall cognitive abilities. On the other hand, N3 sleep seems to improve bodily functions; growth hormones are produced during this stage of sleep, and what happens during this period can have implications on muscle growth and repair of the damages that occur during daily life.

That was a quick introduction to the various stages of sleep that we experience during a normal night of sleep. However, this information does not answer the fundamental question of *why* do we need sleep? Remember, things once weren't so easy for us humans. In the past there were predators looking to gobble up our ancestors, and having the need to get sleep would really have put them in harm's way. It is clear there must be something *absolutely necessary* about sleep; otherwise, Mother Nature, Evolution, or the Creator would have weeded the need for sleep out of us.

What is it that makes sleep necessary for survival? There is no short answer to this question, as sleep is definitely needed for energy conservation, central nervous system functioning, and physical health,[6] but these do not fully explain what is happening to the brain when we sleep. Fortunately, some discoveries in the last few years have really captured the imagination of those interested in the field, and have helped us to get closer to the truth. One such finding is the discovery of what has been called the glymphatic system. In 2013, Dr. Maiken Nedergaard and her colleagues at the University of Rochester Medical Center discovered a system in the brain that drains waste products.[7] Prior to this, it was not known how the brain removes the by-products of daily nerve cell life. All cells require oxygen to survive, and they produce waste products as a result—carbon dioxide, for example. In the brain, there are special waste products that, if not removed, could lead to serious problems over many years, including Alzheimer's disease and Parkinson's disease.

Dr. Nedergaard and her colleagues injected a special dye into the brains of mice and monitored their electrical brain activity, zeroing in on the brain waves we talked about earlier. As reported in the October 18, 2013, edition of *Science*, the dye barely flowed when the mice were awake. In contrast, when the mice were sleeping, especially when in deep (delta wave, slow wave, N3) sleep, it flowed rapidly. It seems that the supporting cells of the brain may actually shrink a little in deep sleep, which then allows the waste products to filter out of the brain.

This new information was groundbreaking for the scientific information itself, but more importantly, it gave us another partial clue as to *why* we sleep—to aid in the removal of waste products. This is a question that has consumed humanity's greatest minds throughout history, and while we are still figuring it out, this research has propelled us forward.

Much more remains to be discovered, but for now, let's continue on our journey and talk about what we do know. On to the next chapter.

3

A NEW PATIENT

When a new patient comes to my office, the first thing I need to know is the reason for the visit. It may be because he or she

- can't get to sleep
- can't stay asleep
- wakes up feeling unrefreshed
- feels tired during the day

This is the kind of overview I need before I can get started. It's the kind I recently got from a patient I'll call Audrey. She presents a fascinating history.

> For the past twelve years I've been a communications and business development executive at large risk-management companies. It's a high-energy, active business. I travel 20 percent or more of the time and I have what I'd describe as a busy, stressful life.
>
> I've been a solid sleeper all my life, including as a child and certainly as a teenager when my parents would tell me it was time to get up because I'd been asleep for eighteen hours.
>
> I don't recall having had any difficulties until early in 2012, when I suddenly realized I was very tired when I woke up in the morning. I had moved to a different company at that point. It involved new work and new responsibilities, plus a lot of stress and anxiety.
>
> The previous winter I had gotten a bad cold and a sinus infection. I couldn't sleep and I assumed that was the main reason I was waking up tired. My doctor gave me what I needed to deal with the cold and

the sinus condition, but he also suggested I might want to see a sleep specialist.

I followed his advice and went to a doctor who sent me home with a vest that was attached to an iPhone that recorded what was going on while I was asleep at night. The results suggested that I had a mild case of obstructive sleep apnea. The doctor explained that this is a condition that blocks the upper airway and causes breathing to stop and start during the night.

The diagnosis helped explain an experience I had a few years earlier. I had an operation in 2009 that required general anesthesia. I was in the recovery room for a long time, not because I wasn't feeling well but because my blood wasn't oxygenating and I kept setting off a buzzer. I overheard the doctor and the nurse talking, and the doctor said she thought I might have obstructive sleep apnea, which would explain why I was nodding off in the recovery room. The nurse said I didn't seem like a candidate for OSA because I wasn't overweight. The doctor said, "True, but sometimes it's hereditary."

Fast-forward to 2012 and the doctor who said I might have sleep apnea also tells me that my tongue sits high in my throat. It could be closing the airway when I fall asleep, he said, and causing me to snore. He also said the OSA could be corrected if I used a CPAP, which is a device that consists of a mask and a hose you wear at night. It supplies a stream of air that keeps the airway in the throat open while you're sleeping. As an alternative, he suggested that I might try propping myself up on pillows when I went to bed.

To the best of my knowledge I wasn't snoring or thrashing around or anything like that, but I asked my husband if he noticed if I stopped breathing during the night. He said not really, but there are times that I snortle and wake up. That was interesting. What the hell is a snortle? He said it's like a hiccup with an oinking sound. It was news to me, but now my husband and I have a new joke about how I snortle myself awake.

It makes sense. My father was a snorer, and one of my three brothers had a terrible snoring problem. He got a new girlfriend at one point and she couldn't stand the snoring. He went to a sleep doctor and he wound up getting a CPAP. It changed their lives and from then on everything was fine.

When I got the diagnosis from my sleep doctor, I figured the snortling was probably my body's way of waking me up and telling me I wasn't breathing. At that point, all the pieces started to fit together. My blood was not oxygenating after my operation, maybe because of my high tongue. And because of the sleep apnea, I wasn't getting enough rest or enough deep sleep, which explained why I felt tired when I woke up.

I was in my fifties then. I did some serious research and concluded I didn't want to go to bed with a machine. I had seen my brother's CPAP. He's very dedicated to it. It's small and he carries it with him when he travels. It's also expensive and takes a lot of maintenance. It's also noisy. I knew my husband wouldn't like that part. I didn't like the part about having to wear a mask to bed and waking up with lines on my face. Not very scientific but I'm a woman and I'm vain.

So I started looking around for other answers. I haven't cured my sleep apnea and I haven't totally stopped the snortling, but since 2012 I have been using a combination of things that are really helping. The most important is an app I discovered for my iPhone called Sleep Cycle. You plug into it when you get in bed and it records everything you do during the night.

It reminds me of the food journal you keep when you're on a diet. You have no trouble remembering that you had a salad and a piece of chicken for dinner, but you tend to forget about the ten pretzels and the four pieces of chocolate and the bag of potato chips you ate during the afternoon. Next thing you know, you add up the calories in the journal and it's far in excess of what you remember and what you're shooting for.

By journaling my sleep, I became aware of how badly I was sleeping and how many times I was getting up during the night. It was obvious why I didn't feel rested when I woke up in the morning. I'm not sure what kind of algorithms the Sleep Cycle uses, but I could suddenly see the number of cycles of deep sleep I was getting each night, the length of time I was actually in bed, and other things of that nature.

What was also clear was the fact that I had no real game plan when it came to sleeping. One of my friends suggested a wellness center. I went to one and learned about meditation and that my body has rhythms I didn't know about. If I want to get quality sleep, it doesn't really have much to do with how much time I spend in bed. It's mainly about those rhythms and about getting up at the same time each morning.

So I changed my sleep habits. We used to watch TV at eleven o'clock but now we record the news and watch it the next morning while we're getting dressed. I'm in bed before 11 and I usually get up around 6:30. Thanks in part to the app, I'm now getting about seven and a half hours of sleep.

We also did a bunch of other things. We got new pillows. My husband and I like ones that are soft and we punch them down before we go to sleep. There was a period of time recently when we just weren't sleeping. We were complaining about the pillows, and I accused my husband of taking my pillow and he said I had taken his. We got a good laugh out of that, but it also sent us in a new direction. We collected all our pillows and, between our bedroom, the kids' room, and the guest room, we realized we had about a dozen really bad pillows.

Over the years I'd go to one of the big stores in the mall and buy pillows for $2.99 and $4.99. After we used them for a few weeks, they became flat as a paper towel. They weren't doing what they should to support us at night. So we found an upscale store that sold pillows that have great names like DreamSleep. We didn't spring for the $150 ones but we bought two new ones for $80 each. They are a combination of old school and new school, some polyester and some feathers. They're punchable and they provide the support I need for reading and sleeping.

After two days with the new pillows we're like, how stupid could we have been that we didn't invest in good pillows earlier in our lives? They've made a huge difference. So now we go to bed at 11 every night. We've got good pillows, and I sleep with my head elevated. When I travel I bring a down jacket that I put under my pillow for extra support.

I use the Sleep Cycle app every night, and it tells me exactly when I go to bed, when I wake up and go to the bathroom, how long I'm up and reading if I can't get back to sleep, how much I've exercised during the day as determined by the number of steps I have taken, how my heart rate correlates with my sleep, and so forth and so on.

If I had a severe case of sleep apnea I'd probably go for more serious stuff, but the things I'm doing seem to be working. I'm sleeping much better. I'm snortling less. And I wake up feeling rested.

Audrey's story is not exactly typical of patients who have sleep problems, but she provides a wonderful history that gives us a lot to think about. Here are a few specifics that jumped out at me:

- Patients often ask where their obstructive sleep apnea (OSA) came from. The fact that Audrey's father and a brother have OSA speaks to how this condition may be inherited to some degree. All three probably have "tight" airways, based on what is known as a *Mallampati*score—the higher the score the tighter the airway.
- To this point, being thin does not mean that a person will not have OSA. The tongue and the soft tissue in the back of the throat are the main issues, as Audrey discovered.
- If you undergo a procedure in which you are anesthetized and you seem to stop breathing in the recovery room, it definitely pays to look into it. The anesthesia may bring OSA to light by relaxing the upper airway muscles further, and having oxygen monitored closely in that setting can reveal the problem.
- Sometimes the bed partner denies any kind of breathing pauses, but when pressed, he or she will report strange noises. We definitely take a bed partner's report seriously, but many times the bed partner, being asleep, does not realize what is happening to the patient. So if the bed partner says, "Yes, I hear breathing pauses," that will aid us, but the lack of that kind of report does not necessarily deter us from testing.
- When a person with Audrey's history uses a firm pillow to provide an incline when sleeping, gravity has less of an effect on pulling the tongue and soft tissue toward the back of her throat, which tightens the airway and causes snoring. This is not always a solution, but it's a route I recommend in mild cases of OSA or when other options are not viable or desired by the patient.
- I don't recommend any particular brands of pillows—or mattresses, for that matter—but I will say this: both the pillow and mattress should be firm enough to support one's head, neck, and spine in an aligned manner. The best position to sleep in is the fetal position, and a firm pillow and mattress can aid in this.
- CPAP (which stands for continuous positive airway pressure) consists of a mask and hose device, worn at nighttime, which sends pressurized air through the nasal passages alone, or through the nasal passages and mouth, down to the back of the throat. It prevents the tongue and the soft tissues from falling down and clogging the airway. We talk about this later in chapter 6, "Obstructive Sleep Apnea."

- I fully realize (and let my patients know) that it is totally under-standable to feel that CPAP will be uncomfortable and daunting at first, but the good news is that it works. A large amount of medical literature shows just how effective it is. However, people may still have valid concerns about marks on their face from a CPAP mask, or other issues such as claustrophobia. If the OSA is mild or moderate, we can often opt for less invasive treatments, such as a mandibular advancement device (MAD). Chapter 6 will have much more information on this issue

- As for the expense issue, insurance carriers typically cover the cost of the entire CPAP unit as well as replacement masks and sup-plies.

- I personally wouldn't base a treatment on sleep apps at this time, but it's clear they are here to stay. They can be fun and easy to use. They also engage the patient in their health and cause them to pay attention to the factors involved in getting quality sleep. Please see chapter 12 for more information on sleep technology.

- Audrey has done a great job making lifestyle/behavioral changes, which in many cases are the most difficult to do. When successful, they can lead to the longest-lasting improvement. I may recom-mend other types of treatment at some point, but Audrey is doing a great job and should keep it up. Please note: she is doing it all without medications.

As I said at the start, the first thing we need to know about a new patient is whether it's a question of getting to sleep, staying asleep, waking up feeling unrefreshed, or feeling tired during the day. Depend-ing on the answer, we move on to finding a solution.

If the problem is getting to sleep, it could be that the patient simply needs a little guidance in terms of sleep hygiene, which we look at in chapter 4, "Insomnia." It could result from anxiety and conditioning, which we also discuss in the next chapter.

If the problem is staying asleep, that opens a host of different pos-sibilities. Difficulty staying asleep may be caused by physical abnormal-ities, including breathing stoppages during the night (typically obstruc-tive sleep apnea, or OSA, which we discuss in chapter 6) or abnormal movements during the night (see chapter 8, on restless legs syndrome, and chapter 9, on the other parasomnias) or even pain. There could be mental problems, including anxiety, stress, or depression, which often cause early morning awakening. There could also be other health issues.

If the patient is not feeling rested throughout the day, it could be because of any one of these issues. It also could be due to a completely separate disorder like narcolepsy. (See chapter 10 for a detailed discussion.)

Bedtime routines and sleep habits are key facts I need to know when I see new patients. I need to know what time they get home from work, when they exercise, and what time they start to wind down. What are they doing in the hours leading up to bed? Are they watching TV? If so, for how long? What time do they eat dinner? What time do they actually get into bed?

Then I'll move on and ask, once they get into bed, typically how long does it take to fall asleep? Are they watching TV or talking with their spouse in bed? Are they on the phone or playing video games in bed?

Sleep latency refers to how long it takes from the time someone turns off the lights to the time they fall asleep. More than half an hour can be problematic, and it may be a sign of what is known as sleep onset insomnia. If this is the problem, I'll ask what they have been doing to deal with it. Most often it's medications that doctors have prescribed or over-the-counter products like melatonin, Benadryl or Benadryl-like substances, Advil PM, Tylenol PM, or other products of this nature. I'll ask if any drug has been effective and, if yes, why they stopped taking it.

I also need to know what happens once they have fallen asleep. Do they wake up during the night? If so, how often? While the number of times could be an issue, I'm more interested in whether they are able to get back to sleep once they wake up. If someone says they wake up once during the night to go to the bathroom and then get right back to sleep, it shouldn't be a problem. If, however, the person wakes up several times during the night and feels fatigued during the day, that could be a whole different story.

I also want to know what the bed partner has to say about what the patient does during the night. In the breathing realm, that could be snoring, gasping for air, choking, or the like. I need to know about arm movements, leg movements, tossing/turning, falling out of bed, rolling from side to side, knocking the sheets off, and putting the bed in disarray. I like to know about talking in their sleep, acting out dreams, striking the bed partner or sleepwalking.

Sleep paralysis, which describes a condition during which someone wakes up abruptly and is not able to move, is another area I need to explore. Patients who experience sleep paralysis are able to move their eyes but cannot move their body. It is typically benign, but if it occurs frequently it may be associated with sleep conditions like obstructive sleep apnea or narcolepsy.

I need to know if new patients have had auditory or visual hallucinations when they are drifting off to sleep or as they are waking up—something like a knocking at the door when no one is really there, or seeing a shape move out of the corner of their eye. Again, these tend to be benign when they occur every now and then. When frequent, they could be markers of certain sleep conditions, most notably narcolepsy. The term for them is *hypnagogic* hallucinations if they occur when someone is falling asleep, or *hypnopompic* hallucinations when they are waking up.

Once I discover what's happening when a person sleeps, I'll want to know about the wake-up time on weekdays and weekends. If someone is very consistent during the week—sleeping, say, from 11 p.m. to 7 a.m.—and then going to bed at 3 a.m. and waking up at 1 p.m. on weekends, that could be a problem, particularly for those suffering with insomnia. Additionally, I may inquire *why* they feel they have to sleep late; is it because they are sleep deprived during the week?

I want to know if my patients set an alarm. Do they doze off when it rings? And how do they feel throughout the day? Are they exhausted when they get out of bed? Does it take a couple of hours to fully wake up? Once into the day, are they dozing on the train on the way to work or on the way home? Are they falling asleep in traffic? At a red light? How are they at work? How is their mood? How much coffee are they drinking?

To help put this information into perspective, I ask my patients to fill out an *Epworth Sleepiness Scale*, which is basically a subjective measure of how sleepy someone is throughout the day. And then, of course, I want to know about the other medical problems they have that might be causing the sleep issues that brought them to me.

Once we understand what the problem is, we can begin to focus on the solution—and, as with all aspects of medicine, there is no one right approach for everyone. I first may try to figure out if there are simple things to do, such as an improvement in sleep habits, before we have to either prescribe or change medications or if we need to do a sleep test to come up with additional information.

When we ask someone to come in for an overnight sleep test (it's called a polysomnogram, or PSG), it's generally because of a suspicion of obstructive sleep apnea, restless legs syndrome, or periodic leg movements during sleep. It could be a suspicion of a parasomnia, which is a condition like sleepwalking. We may suspect narcolepsy. Or it could be we are just not really sure what's happening when the patient falls asleep.

Overnight sleep tests vary from place to place, but the patient generally arrives between 8 p.m. and 10 p.m., and then gets "hooked-up," which takes about forty-five minutes. Electrodes are attached to the patient's scalp with an electro-paste or conductive paste. The electrodes allow us to monitor brain waves, which tell us whether the person is actually sleeping or awake, and what stage of sleep he or she is in. For a look at how this all works, a Google search of "polysomnogram" will turn up a number of good photos of people actually undergoing an overnight test.

We also monitor the airflow and the respiratory effort to determine if someone is having obstructive or central sleep apnea. We do a limited EKG, which looks at the heart rhythm. We read the blood oxygen level. We do muscle monitoring through an electrode near the chin. Other electrodes on the shins measure foot flexing and foot movement throughout the night. There can be more tests and more electrodes if we see the need for them, but that's the standard setup.

A patient will often ask me, "How am I going to sleep with all this equipment covering every part of my body?" I'm honest about it and I tell them it's not going to be the best night of their life. But even if the patient only sleeps for a few hours, it usually gives us the information we need. If we're looking for sleep apnea or suspect movements during the night, a few hours will usually be enough for a good diagnosis. The majority of people say they woke up several times during the test and didn't feel like they slept much, but in most cases we come away with enough information. It's very rare that we have a truly failed test.

Another question patients ask is what happens if they have to get up during the night to go to the bathroom. That's an easy one. The electrodes are all attached to an electronic box, and the box is attached to a wall unit. Our technical people are on the scene during the night, and if a patient says he or she needs to go to the bathroom, someone will come in and detach the electrodes. The box remains around the person's neck in the bathroom. Upon returning, the box is hooked back into the wall unit and the test resumes.

The patient wakes up in the morning, gets unhooked, uses the shower if he or she chooses to, and then heads home. Once all the data are collected and scored, the patient receives a full report from the physician and we move on from there.

In some cases of excessive sleepiness or fatigue, when the likelihood of sleep apnea or other physical sleep issues are not suspected, we look at the possibility of narcolepsy and its cousin, idiopathic hypersomnia. To diagnose these conditions, we perform an additional test, an MSLT, or Multiple Sleep Latency Test, which is basically a nap test. We discuss this in chapter 10.

Given the insurance environment these days, in-lab sleep tests are not always approved by medical insurance carriers. One option is a sleep test at home, which is a viable path if the problem appears to be simple OSA. The home test measures airflow (via a sensor in the nose and mouth), the breathing effort (a belt around the chest), and oxygen levels (an oximeter on the finger). These tests do not measure actual sleep time, nor do they account for other problems that may occur, so they may underestimate the depth of some sleep issues. But for simple OSA, an in-home test is a reasonable alternative.

Once the information from the sleep test is combined with the data from the patient's history, we move on to a treatment plan, which is the focus of the next chapters.

SUMMARY AND ACTION PLAN

Before going to see a sleep specialist, it's a good idea to compile a list of information that will give the doctor a picture of what is going on in your life and provide background before a treatment plan is actually created. The following information should be organized, if not on paper, at least in your mind:

- Your sleep schedule—the time you go to bed during the week and on weekends, and your typical bedtime habits.

- A bed partner's report of what you do while you are asleep—snoring, gasping, moving, talking, and walking around are important pieces of the puzzle that should be shared with the doctor.
- Note the times you nap or doze off during a typical week and how long you sleep.
- A list of the medications, over-the-counter products, and the various treatments you have tried to deal with your sleep problems, along with data on the ones that have helped and the ones that haven't.
- A list of the substances you take during the day—alcohol, tobacco, nicotine, and any illicit drugs—and when you take them.
- A copy of any sleep tests or relevant blood tests you have had.
- A talk with family members (Mom, Dad, and siblings) about the sleep problems they may be dealing with, or have dealt with, including even seemingly mild things like snoring.

4

INSOMNIA

"**T**he patient should wake during the day and sleep during the night." These words come from Hippocrates, the Greek physician who is considered one of the most outstanding figures in the history of medicine. He had lots to say about sleep and sleeplessness, including this: "The worst part is to get no sleep either night or day, for it follows from this symptom that the insomnolency is connected with sorrow and pains, or that he is about to become delirious."

Insomnia is the name for a condition in which a person can't get to sleep, can't stay sleep, or has unrefreshing sleep. As you can guess from what Hippocrates told us, insomnia (or, as he referred to it, "insomnolency") can be extremely distressing, both in its acute and chronic types. Let's take a look at both.

Acute insomnia is usually due to anxiety-provoking events that everyone has experienced. The night before a big test, a big game, or a big presentation, many of us simply cannot sleep. This is due to the activation of the central nervous system's defense mechanism, generally known as the "fight-or-flight" response.

Imagine a caveman in his camp, surrounded by a pack of wild animals. His biggest worry is whether a lion, tiger, or bear is going to eat him or his family. Do you think it would be wise for him to be deeply asleep in that situation, or asleep at all, knowing that at any minute a beast could find him and his family and turn them into a midnight snack?

Obviously not, which is why nature armed human beings with the ability to stave off the need for sleep and ramp up the fight-or-flight response in times of danger. In the event that a bear comes within attacking distance, it would be helpful to not only not be asleep but also to be "wired" and ready to run if the situation deems it necessary.

Fortunately, in our modern times, most of us don't have to worry about bears or other wild animals coming into our bedrooms and attacking us, but in the case of insomnia, the reaction we have is the same. One such response would be hypervigilance, which is basically having a heightened sense of noise or movement. Being hypervigilant when it is time for bed makes sleep extremely difficult. Regular everyday noises can startle the insomniac and cause him or her to jump at the slightest sound, keeping the person up and even more alert and awake.

Acute insomnia usually is self-limited, meaning that once the stressor is removed (i.e., the big test is over) sleeping patterns return to normal. Some physicians choose to treat this kind of insomnia with medications. People who know that they get like this before a big day can ask their doctor to prescribe an anxiolytic or a hypnotic, which are fancy names for types of sleeping pills.

When the problem involves more than just a few nights in a row, we call it *chronic insomnia* (by definition, insomnia that occurs at least three nights per week over a period of at least three months). Dr. Art Spielman, a colleague of mine who sadly passed away a few years ago, developed what he called the 3P model of chronic insomnia, which is a way of understanding where the insomnia comes from.[1] The first P stands for "predisposing," which would be something like a family history of insomnia or a personal history of anxiety or panic. The second P is for "precipitating," which could be something like a divorce, a death in the family, or a job change, at which point the predisposition that was lying dormant becomes active. The third P is for "perpetuating" factors like bad sleep habits, spending too much time in bed, and seeing bed as a place of stress rather than a place of sleep. When these three Ps become a problem, sleep becomes a problem.

The last P in this mode, "perpetuating," is where sleep hygiene comes into play. What is sleep hygiene, you may ask? It's not how clean your bed is—rather, it is a measure of how sleep inducing one's bedroom and bedroom practices are. Improving sleep hygiene is imperative for dealing with insomnia.

With this in mind, let's take a look at what Myra, a patient of mine, has to say about her experiences with chronic insomnia.

I have never been a great sleeper, but my real troubles started twenty-three years ago when my first child was born. I needed to be at the ready in terms of getting up and tending to her, feeding her, and taking care of her, and from that point on I became a very light sleeper. I didn't do anything about it for about twenty years. I had one child and then a second and a third, but it wasn't until about four years ago that I realized I was exhausted all the time and that I had a sleep issue that should and probably could be addressed.

I had no problem falling asleep, but most nights I would wake up around two and then be totally awake for two or more hours. I'd fall back to sleep around four or five in the morning, but then I'd have to get up at six and that was hard. I have a busy New York City life, and I was exhausted much of the day. One of the turning points came when I recognized what my sleep problem was doing to me: I would dash home from work every day, put dinner on the table for my family, and then collapse.

At that point, I started seeing a new internist. She asked all kinds of basic questions and then asked about my sleep patterns. When I was leaving, she gave me a printout with a list of dos and don'ts. She said that 90 percent of the people who do everything suggested in the printout sleep through the night. They were things like absolutely no caffeine, no alcohol, going to bed at the same time every night, and getting exercise five times a week. It was a good list, but it didn't help me. I already did 100 percent of the things on the list.

One of my friends suggested a Qi Gong class, which is a Chinese movement–type program. The man who ran it said it would help me sleep. It didn't. Somewhere along the way a neighbor told me about a mindfulness meditation workshop called "How to Get a Good Night's Sleep." I Googled it and it looked good. According to the promotional material, if you meditate forty-five minutes a day, you will supposedly get a good night's sleep after eight weeks or so. I couldn't attend the workshop because of my schedule, but I signed up for an individual class and began a mindfulness-based stress reduction program.

At about the same time, I started seeing Dr. Barone. After a few visits, he asked me to spend a night at the Weill Cornell Center for Sleep Medicine. My face, heart, and legs were hooked up to electrodes. It wasn't horrendous, but it was uncomfortable, and I couldn't help wondering how I was going to sleep with all this stuff on. I guess I slept, but I remember a great feeling of liberation when I walked out the next morning.

The good news is that I didn't have sleep apnea. Dr. Barone said my pattern of waking up in the middle of the night suggested chronic insomnia. Based on the diagnosis, he prescribed zolpidem at first, then eszopiclone. Neither helped with my sleep issues, and I didn't react well to them. They knocked the stuffing out of my body, but my mind was wide awake, and it was an uncomfortable feeling. I also knew they were going to be hard to get off, so I was pleased when Dr. Barone suggested trazodone, which he said is a mild antidepressant that often helps with insomnia.

The trazodone did the trick, but it was only one piece of the puzzle. Dr. Barone would ask me to fill out a questionnaire at the start of each visit that contained a lot of questions—do I fall asleep while I'm sitting in a car or at a movie, for instance, and how many times do I wake up each night. He kept a record of my answers from visit to visit, and seeing the progress I was making was helpful. Slowly but surely I began to sleep better.

Another thing that helped—and it's something I remember to this day whenever I wake in the middle of the night—was that Dr. Barone would always say we're aiming for improvement, not perfection. In other words, we shouldn't focus on how many hours of sleep I'm getting but on how I feel during the day. He also stressed that change wasn't going to happen overnight.

So it was a combination: trazodone; meditation; the understanding that we're looking for improvement, not perfection; realizing that the process would take time; and seeing Dr. Barone and talking things over with him on a regular basis. I now take trazodone regularly and see Dr. Barone every ten months. I visit the stress reduction person once a month. I try to meditate every morning and I meditate in the middle of the night if I wake up.

Things were improving and they got even better when I realized I could improve the odds further if I got to bed earlier, and that's what I've been doing. I now get to bed by 10:30 and stay in bed until about 6:30, and it helps. I still wake up at night but I can usually get back to sleep. The torment is no longer there. I don't have long bouts of staying awake anymore, and that's been a huge plus for me.

I'm fifty-four now. My first daughter was born twenty-three years ago, but the last ten years were the worst in terms of sleeping. By that point, I wasn't getting up to care for babies but a sleep pattern had been entrenched. Things are much better now because of everything I've learned. We're not aiming for perfection, it takes a while for change to happen, and it takes energy and effort. There's no magic pill, despite what the pharmaceutical companies keep telling us. You have to attack the problem from all angles.

Myra gives us a lot to think about. To begin with, her internist was absolutely correct by starting with sleep hygiene improvement. Unfortunately, her case required a bit more, which is not uncommon. Mindfulness meditation, hypnotherapy, acupuncture, and the like can all be extremely helpful things to experiment with. I always tell my patients, *if it doesn't hurt, it's worth a try.*

- As Myra suggests, undergoing an overnight sleep test can be an intimidating experience. But I told her, as I tell all my patients, that the overnight test is not going to be the best night of your life. But even if you just get a few solid hours of sleep, that will usually help me to determine what is at issue. So really you should not stress about it.
- I initially thought zolpidem (Ambien) or eszopiclone (Lunesta) would be helpful for Myra. I tried zolpidem to help improve her ability to fall asleep, which did not work well enough, and then eszopiclone to help her fall and stay asleep, which had similarly unimpressive results. We talked about anxiety/depression as possibly playing a role in her sleep issues, which she agreed with. At that time we tried trazodone and went on from there.
- The questionnaire Myra is referring to is called the Epworth Sleepiness Scale, which is used by clinicians as a subjective tool to monitor how patients feel in the daytime. It is far from perfect, but is a good way to keep track of treatment progress. It consists of eight scenarios in which someone could potentially be drowsy, and the patient is asked to fill out the likelihood (never, rarely, occasionally, frequently) of falling asleep. A score above 8–10 out of a possible 24 is considered being excessively sleepy.
- Sleep is not something that we can "perfect." It may be that some people will never have the full eight continuous hours that we are led to believe is ideal. This is okay. What we should be looking at is how we can improve upon the problem, and focusing on how we feel throughout the day. By not being too concerned with what

is "not right," Myra has been able to improve upon what is right with her sleep.

Another patient, Jordan, has an equally fascinating history that sheds light on other aspects of chronic insomnia.

I'm thirty-nine. I am a management consultant, which can be a stressful job. Stress is one of the problems that brought me to Dr. Barone. It's interrelated with another medical condition I had since I was six or seven years old, which is migraine headaches.

I've had sleep problems all my life, in part because I've always been very sensitive to noise and light. Ever since I was young, I would make sure my bedroom had dark blackout curtains. I would try to minimize noise by putting towels underneath the door and I would always ask my parents to try to keep the noise down so I could sleep.

When I went to middle school, a new element entered my life. I joined the swim team and had to get up early for practice. Sometimes 4:45 in the morning, sometimes 5:15. To get up that early, I needed to go to bed at eight, sometimes nine o'clock at night. In the summertime there usually was a little light still outside, so a lot of time I was trying to go to sleep when my body really wasn't ready for it.

That was the cause of my real issues with sleep. I was getting up very early and trying to force myself to go to bed early so I wouldn't be overtired the next day. I was on the swim team for two years in middle school and then almost all my years in high school. I would get very nervous about approaching sleep because I didn't feel ready to go to bed. I also knew that if I didn't get a good night's sleep, it would impact me negatively the next day in terms of my performance at swim practice and school.

As a result, I developed insomnia. Whenever I have a very stressful day, I have trouble sleeping because I can't turn my mind off. I also have another major problem. I live in New York. I'm exposed to noise that I don't have any control over, and having unpredictable noises gives me a sense of anxiety.

This is where Dr. Barone has made a large impact in my overall sleep quality and my overall level of mental and physical well-being. We determined at the start that I needed to come up with a plan. So I attacked the first item: reducing levels of stress to help my mind shut down, so when it is time to go to bed, I'm able to do it.

I attacked this part of the problem in four ways. First, I now do daily exercise, in particular yoga. I started yoga in 2009, but I never really did it consistently. In the last couple of years I've been doing it five times a week. That's probably had the strongest impact in terms of my overall sleep quality because yoga helps me focus. It makes my mind go blank, especially when I'm sitting quietly before practice starts and then after when it's over. It's been very helpful in training me to let my mind stop running at a frenetic pace and just kind of stop.

The second thing I've been doing is keeping an eye on all my triggers. I used to have one or two drinks after work with friends. I've cut that out. I used to have a cup of coffee in the afternoon. I stopped that. I mentioned migraines earlier. There's some overlap with the triggers for sleep and the triggers for migraines. Cutting back on alcohol and coffee helped reduce my migraines, which has been a nice added benefit. Combined with the yoga, I think it's brought down the severity of my migraines as well as the number of attacks per month.

The third thing I've been doing is watching what I eat. For the last year and a half, I've been cooking the majority of my meals at home. Five or more times per week I've been cooking dinner at home, and I've been having lunch and breakfast at home too. This has had a profound impact on my overall well-being and my sleep quality, in large part because I have a greater understanding of what I'm putting into my body.

I was going through tons of zolpidem in the past. I was trying to go to sleep; it wasn't happening and I didn't have a real plan. I was eating poorly, I wasn't really exercising, and I was letting stress get to me. All these different elements were part of my life, and I needed to get an understanding of what they were and get them under control.

The fourth thing I've been doing to manage stress is something I never really thought about before Dr. Barone mentioned it. I was going to bed at a strict time each night, usually at 11. I'd turn the lights down and get into bed whether I felt sleepy or not. I've totally abandoned that model. I now only go to bed when I start to feel really tired, and sometimes I'll be up until one or two o'clock in the morning. When I start to feel tired, then I'll go to bed. And then I'll give it a good half hour or so to try to let it take hold. If it doesn't, I'll get up and maybe take a little zolpidem as a backstop.

I now only have a handful of times each month when I need to get up and say, okay, I've given sleep half an hour, I've tried to calm my mind, I ate right today, I went to yoga, I did everything right but my body still doesn't want to give itself over to sleep, so I'm going to take 3 mg of zolpidem and call it a night. My overarching goal is to approach sleep without seeing it as some kind of dreaded thing. I can see it as something I have a symbiotic relationship with. It's the psychology of approaching sleep that Dr. Barone has helped me understand. It doesn't have to be an epic battle of me versus the bed.

Another thing: If I've had three nights in a row of good sleep and I have one bad night, I'm not going to let that one bad one get to me. I'm going to say to myself, okay, Jordan, you had three good nights of good sleep and this is a bad night, but if you average them out you're batting 75 percent and that's not that bad. If you batted that in the major leagues you'd be making millions.

While it is often true that insomnia occurs following a major life event, some people like Jordan have insomnia starting at a very young age. The technical name for this is *idiopathic insomnia*, and it can be quite difficult to treat. Sleep and sleep health are closely related with psychological states such as stress, anxiety, and depression. Same with headaches.

- When Jordan was forced to change his sleep habits to meet the demands of the swim team, he was working against his body's internal clock, which is very hard to do. This is where the vicious cycle of insomnia and bedtime anxiety becomes prevalent. The very nature of having insomnia makes people get anxious about bedtime, which worsens the insomnia, and that, in turn, worsens the anxiety. Treating both the anxiety and stress in conjunction with the insomnia is of paramount importance. A lot of times, patients will want the insomnia treated but don't pay enough attention to the anxiety/stress/depression/ruminating thoughts that are driving it. We need to take care of all relevant factors causing the insomnia if we want to improve in a meaningful way.
- People who sleep lightly and have difficulty falling asleep may be bothered by even light noise. A white-noise machine, a fan, or earplugs may be useful.

- Jordan took the stress-reduction plan to heart. Yoga is a wonderful tool to calm the mind, as are regular meditation, acupuncture, Tai Chi, massage therapy, and others. These natural/homeopathic approaches are underutilized for insomnia, which is a shame because they have no side effects and can be incredibly helpful.
- Caffeine and alcohol affect sleep, and Jordan did a great job of reducing their impact. Diet may also impact sleep in that having heavy meals close to bed can lead to sleep disruption. A good diet, along with other healthy lifestyle choices, can be beneficial to overall well-being.
- Zolpidem (Ambien) unfortunately tends to be thought of as a cure-all for insomnia. And while it does have a role when used in the right situation, the job of sleep specialists is to see if there are longer-term solutions to treating insomnia aside from the "quick fix" of medications. The right way to use zolpidem is to take it just as needed and after other approaches have been properly employed.
- Jordan mentions something that's very important here: going to bed only when sleepy is a wonderful tactic that people with insomnia tend not to do. Rather, hoping to get more sleep, they often get into bed when they are not really sleepy. This leads to lying in bed wide awake with ruminating thoughts, frustration, and anxiety, all of which perpetuate the insomnia. Going to bed only when sleepy, even when it is later in the night, can be a really helpful sleep hygiene technique.
- Having a positive outlook about the bed and sleep environment can have a big impact on sleep. This is important in the reconditioning plan of improving sleep hygiene. A lot of times insomnia results from the brain having been "conditioned" to think of bed as a place of stress or anxiety. Now that Jordan gets into bed only when sleepy and does all of the other good sleep techniques, his bed has become a "friendly place" in his mind, and this allows him to sleep easier.
- With his new approach, Jordan has reduced the pressure to fall asleep and has made it easier on himself. While not used by us in this case, some clinicians employ a sleep hygiene technique known as paradoxical intention. This is when we tell patients to say to themselves, "I want to stay awake, I want to stay awake, I

want to stay awake," which usually has the opposite effect. It helps them sleep by reducing the "performance anxiety" that comes with being anxious about insomnia and falling asleep.

- I sometimes see myself as a coach in a sense that I encourage patients to stick with the plan even if there are bad nights. I warn them that there are going to be ups and downs with insomnia, as it does have a waxing and waning nature, but that we are in it together and we will make it work.

As it should be clear by now, insomnia has different causes and there are different approaches to treating it.

Treating chronic insomnia can be done effectively with a combination of techniques known as cognitive behavioral therapy for insomnia,[2] abbreviated as CBT-I. CBT-I is a collection of advanced practices used by clinicians to help retrain the brain to understand that the bed is for sleep.

While historically CBT-I has been a technique done with the help of a specialist, Internet-based CBT-I programs have recently come on the market. One brand, SHUTi, uses similar approaches that a sleep expert would, but they are done in a computer-based format in which the techniques are taught to consumers who use them and track improvement over time. Some data[3] suggest these approaches can be an effective solution for chronic insomnia. As with all relatively new treatments, however, it is not the first thing we usually recommend.

With that in mind, let's go over two of the most important CBT-I techniques, *sleep restriction therapy* and *stimulus control therapy*.

Sleep restriction therapy doesn't sound like a fun time, but it can be a very effective treatment. I absolutely recommend that this technique be done under the guidance of a sleep specialist, and you will see why.

The easiest way to explain how it works is through an extreme example. Let's say a person gets into bed at 8 p.m. but doesn't fall asleep until midnight. Then midnight comes along and he's waking up every hour, and then he finally gets out of bed at 8 a.m. He's in bed from 8 p.m. to 8 a.m., twelve hours, but let's say he's only sleeping six.

Why is this a problem? When people spend too much time in bed, their brain starts to get conditioned. In effect, it says, "This bed is not my place of sleep. This is my place of worry. This is my place of frustration. This is my place of anxiety." On and on and on. And then, as the nights run into each other, it becomes very hard to fall asleep.

What we want to do in this case is actually retrain the brain, and we do it via sleep restriction. I'll tell a patient not to get into bed until 1 a.m. and then to wake up at 7 a.m. It's not meant to be punishing, but what it means is that the patient can only sleep a maximum of six hours at night.

Over a period of a few weeks, the patient's brain begins to restructure itself. It "knows" that it is only allowed six hours in bed, so it has to "make the most" of the time it is given. Patients will go through several days of being sleep deprived, and likely being tired through the day. To make it worse, I tell them they cannot nap. Over a few weeks, the brain begins to say, "My bed is for sleep and that's what I do there." The first couple of weeks are hell. Most of the time my patients are cursing my name, but sleep restriction therapy usually works if they stick to it.

While this can be incredibly effective, there are possible risks. People with bipolar disorder, for example, may actually be induced into a full-blown manic episode as a result of sleep restriction. I can't stress enough that a sleep specialist needs to be involved when anyone decides to try sleep restriction therapy.

The other technique, stimulus control therapy, harkens back to the age-old rule of only using the bed for sleep and sex. Here's how it works. Let's say someone gets into bed at 11 p.m. and cannot get to sleep. Twenty minutes has gone by, and it's obvious sleep is not going to happen. Instead of lying there ruminating and feeling frustrated, I suggest that the person get up out of bed, go to another area of the house—the living room, wherever—and do a relaxing activity.

This can be mindfulness meditation (my favorite one, as we discussed in chapter 1), reading a book on paper, listening to an audio book or soft music, a warm bath, sitting quietly with some candles—and so on. The principle here is to relax without utilizing the electronic devices we have come to rely on. In fact, the TV, tablet, computer, smartphone, and all aspects of the work environment should definitely be out of the bedroom or at least out of the bed space.

Once people are feeling more relaxed, they can get back into bed and try again. And doing this as many times as it takes, while certainly frustrating in the beginning, can be effective long term.

The important thing to remember is that we are retraining the brain to look at the bed and bedroom as the place of sleep, not of stress, worry, and similar problems. It's a message that got through to Marlene, another patient who has a fascinating history.

I'm sixty-one years old, married, and the mother of two. I am a health care administrator who works in risk management and patient safety. For fifteen to twenty years I'd go to sleep at eight or nine o'clock, wake up sometime around midnight or one in the morning, and then toss and turn for the rest of the night. I never got a full night's sleep. I repeated this pattern for many years.

I'm a big tea drinker, and I would try "remedies" like chamomile tea or whatever sleep teas I'd come across. I'd get extra-strength Sleepytime Tea, and use two bags. Whatever I thought would be helpful.

I also did some mindfulness meditation training, and it helped intermittently. Then, in late 2012, I attended a health seminar, and one of the speakers gave a very engaging talk about the harmful effects of sleep deprivation. It made me sit up and take notice. Some of the problems she described were things I was experiencing. My blood pressure was beginning to increase, and I was having all sorts of related problems. She also talked about the public health dangers of sleep deprivation. The realization that I could be putting other people at risk scared me.

I decided it was time to see a sleep specialist. My first doctor was very "by the book." Once he got a sense of my sleep situation, he said the way to deal with it was to stay up till midnight and get up at 5:30 a.m. I disliked his approach intensely. Sitting up and waiting for midnight was torture.

Then I saw Dr. Barone, who took a very different approach. He taught me the elements of cognitive behavioral therapy. I'm not a television watcher, but I used to read in bed, and I discovered this was not the best thing to do. I never used an alarm to wake up. I do now, and it's a big help. Dr. Barone incorporated what I already knew about meditation into my sleep preparation. I had to have a definitive sleep time and specific preparations leading up to it so my body would know I was preparing to go to sleep. This was hugely important.

He told me that he could offer medication, but I was dead set against it and he did not push it. He agreed that if I could do it without being medicated, my sleep would be better. But then I came across valerian tea, and he did not pooh-pooh it. He showed me how I could incorporate herbal teas into my treatment. He had me keep sleep logs and he would add small amounts of time to my sleep goal.

It has made an incredible difference in my life. All those years I'd say to myself, "Listen, you're a tough kid, just tough it out." But it didn't work. Maybe I don't need to sleep much, but who wants to lie awake for four or five hours?

I also learned that if I wasn't able to go back to sleep within a half hour or so, I should get up and do something else. That was something that never occurred to me, and I didn't relish the idea. Some nights now I may wake up two or three times, but they are few and far between. And if I do, I'm able to get back to sleep. There are many nights when I don't wake up at all. I get up most days feeling well rested and ready for whatever lies ahead.

One of the methods I use to help me get to sleep is progressive muscle relaxation. I also use a device that tracks my sleep activity, and from time to time I use melatonin, which is a natural substance. I take 5 mg about an hour before I want to go to sleep. I also use a lamp in the morning to simulate sunlight.

If I had to name three things that are most important, they'd be a consistent bedtime; the use of an alarm, which I always thought was a crutch; and an overall appreciation for the importance of sleep.

Over-the-counter remedies like Sleepytime Tea may be of help for some people, but more aggressive strategies may be needed for others, especially in situations like Marlene's case, where she had been suffering for years and years. Other points that merit repeating:

- Sleep problems can have real consequences to one's own health, as well as to the health of others. A case in point: drowsy driving.
- Sleep restriction can be a powerful technique, but it's not for everyone.
- Marlene succeeded in part because she did a great job of creating and sticking to the plan she developed. She has an open mind. I find this to be incredibly important because some of the things we do to treat insomnia may seem counterintuitive.
- I am not against medications per se, but if we can improve sleep without it, that is best.
- Using sleep logs can be helpful for both doctor and patient to examine their progress in a more objective fashion. The sleep logs

I prefer can be found at the American Academy of Sleep Medicine's website: http://yoursleep.aasmnet.org/pdf/sleepdiary.pdf.

- Some people can do fine on five hours of sleep, but they are truly a rarity.

- When Marlene is talking about progressive muscle relaxation, she is referring to a process by which a person contracts and then relaxes each muscle group, going from head to toe, over a period of fifteen minutes or so. Actively contracting and relaxing each muscle group can help relax both body and mind; if interested, there are many great (and free) resources to be found online.

- Marlene gives us a really nice overview of what stimulus control therapy is all about. I wanted her to use the bed for sleep and nothing else. Therefore, when she is not sleeping, she finds a way to relax elsewhere, until she is ready to fall back asleep.

- In the case of melatonin, I usually recommend 1 mg to 3 mg (either in pill or liquid form), but in some people we may go to 5 mg or higher. What Marlene has done with the lamp in the morning is "trick" her brain into shutting off her own melatonin production to aid in waking her up. Taking melatonin at bedtime and using sunlight or bright light in the morning can be a huge help in regulating one's internal clock.

Even with the approaches Myra, Jordan, and Marlene have adopted, chronic insomnia may take a fair amount of time before it gets better, and we may need to add a sleeping pill.

Medications and substances that help people sleep can be broken down into several categories:

- The benzodiazepine drugs (sometimes referred to as "benzos"), including alprazolam (Xanax), clonazepam (Klonopin), lorazepam (Ativan), and diazepam (Valium). These are medications that help the brain and body relax. They are usually used in the psychiatric realm to reduce anxiety, panic attacks, and the like.

- The so-called non-benzodiazepine drugs (the "non-benzos") like eszopiclone (Lunesta), zolpidem (Ambien), and zaleplon (Sonata). Known as the "Z" drugs, they are what we call non-benzodiazepine receptor agents, which activate the benzodiazepine receptors in the brain without actually being benzodiazepine drugs. They don't relax the muscles or reduce anxiety as much as benzodiaze-pine drugs, but they do have a sleep-inducing effect.

- Melatonin-based medications, such as over-the-counter melato-nin pills and ramelteon (Rozerem), are effective in some cases. We will talk more about melatonin very soon (chapter 5).
- Suvorexant (Belsomra), which has an entirely different way of working compared to the others, basically shuts off the wake-promoting substances in the brain to produce sleep.
- Others include antidepressants like trazodone or doxepin, or an antipsychotic like quetiapine (Seroquel), which tends be used off-label.
- Advil PM, Tylenol PM, and other over-the-counter preparations like Benadryl contain diphenhydramine, which is an antihistamine that causes sleepiness.
- And finally there are natural preparations like cherry extract, va-lerian, and others (see the next chapter).

While there are always risks to anything we put in our bodies, the main things to look out for with these medications and substances is dizziness or feeling hungover the next day. With the benzos there are risks of addiction. With both the benzos and the non-benzos there is a possibility of obstructive sleep apnea (OSA) becoming worse on the nights they are taken. Even with the natural substances, I strongly ad-vise consulting a doctor before starting any of the over-the-counter or herbal preparations.

One thing I like to mention to my patients is that the components of some over-the-counter substances like ibuprofen (Advil PM, for exam-ple), acetaminophen (Tyenol PM, for example), and others can affect the liver over time. It is not good to take them often if they are not needed. If someone were to use one of them, it's best to stick with the "PM" component, which is diphenhydramine (another name for the well-known antihistamine Benadryl). That said, both the medical litera-ture and my clinical experience clearly suggest that diphenhydramine is not great as a sleep aid.

There are several reasons for this, the most glaring being that it can leave us feeling hungover the next day, regardless of how much or how well we slept. Additionally, we habituate to diphenhydramine very quickly, which means that after using the same dose for a couple of weeks, patients may find that they need higher and higher doses to achieve the same effect. In the case of a cold or other short-lived problem, "PM" preparations are okay to use, but I certainly would not rely on them for anything more than just a couple of nights.

The best way to choose what medication to use is a complicated process and hinges upon several factors. First, we need to determine if this is a problem falling asleep, staying asleep, or both. Certain medications are better than others for each. Second, is the patient taking other medications that could interact with the proposed pill? Third, have other issues been properly addressed? For example, if someone has OSA and is waking up in the middle of the night because of stoppages of breathing, zolpidem may not be the best choice. Rather, treating the OSA and seeing how that improves the insomnia would be the preferable way to go. Then, if the patient is still waking in the middle of the night, a course of zolpidem may be totally appropriate.

I can't tell you how important anxiety and depression are when it comes to insomnia. Many patients who come to me because they can't sleep don't actually have a "sleep problem." They may, in fact, be suffering with either or both of these. Classically, anxiety may cause problems falling asleep and depression often causes early morning awakening. I can help these people and work with them, but in many cases an evaluation by a therapist or a psychiatrist would be really helpful.

Certain substances may cause or worsen insomnia. For example, nicotine is a stimulant, which means smoking even a couple hours before bed can lead to difficulty with sleep. Diet pills can often stimulate the body, again making it difficult to fall or stay asleep. Similarly, caffeine can last a while in the body (even hours after the energy boost wears off) and can therefore make it more difficult to fall asleep.

Finally, people will frequently tell me that a glass of wine with dinner or right before bed helps them to sleep. What's interesting is that after falling asleep with alcohol in the system, the first hour or so will usually be okay. But alcohol is a depressant, and once it is metabolized the body responds in a reverse way. In other words, one may go from being in a relaxed state to suddenly waking up sweating, with a dry mouth, or needing to urinate. Furthermore, it can worsen snoring and OSA, also leading to awakenings through the night. Bottom line: It's not a good idea to rely on alcohol for insomnia.

SUMMARY AND ACTION PLAN

To reiterate, when we talk about sleep hygiene, we are talking about a collection of practices needed to have normal, high-quality sleep, along with daytime alertness. Improving sleep hygiene is probably the best way to go when it comes to an initial plan to combat insomnia.

- The easiest place to start would be to shut off electronic devices that have a backlit screen thirty to sixty minutes before sleep time, and certainly not to use them in bed or if you wake in the middle of the night.
- Use the bed and bedroom only for sleep and sex. If you have to do anything in bed aside from these, try reading a book or magazine on paper for fifteen to twenty minutes, or listening to soft music.
- Keep a strict sleep-wake schedule. This is important especially on the weekends when many people "sleep in." This can throw off your internal clock.
- Get regular exercise, ideally in the morning.
- Avoid caffeine after 1–2 p.m.
- Eliminate nicotine and reduce alcohol, especially close to bedtime.
- Getting sunlight in the morning can be useful to teach your brain that this is the time to be awake. I recommend twenty minutes or so, not to get a tan but to get your brain to shut off melatonin and really wake itself up.
- Drink water throughout the day, but a couple hours before bedtime would be a good time to stop.
- Practice relaxation techniques, such as mindfulness meditation, regularly.

Improving sleep hygiene is a start, but there are other treatments:

- Behavioral modification: stimulus control therapy, sleep restriction therapy.
- Medications: benzo drugs, non-benzo drugs, and others.
- The literature shows that while medications may have the best track record on a short-term basis, behavioral modification wins out over the long term.
- A combination approach is probably most effective overall.

5

DOING WHAT COMES NATURALLY

Many of my patients ask me about natural remedies that they can try to help with insomnia. I am a fan of things that *may* be helpful, and ideally are not likely to be harmful. Supplements I sometimes recommend include melatonin, valerian root, magnesium, cherry extract, passionflower, and several others. In general they are safe, but a doctor should be told when you are taking them, since there can be interactions with medications.

Natural remedies fall into a category similar to vitamins. That means they are not covered by Federal Drug Administration (FDA) regulations, so the purity of one company's pill may not be the same as another's. That being the case, I always suggest buying from a reputable source.

As for the hard science behind them, I regret to say that in rigorous studies comparing the natural substances to a placebo, not a great deal of data emerge that show their efficacy. At the same time, some data suggest that they may actually be harmful. Valerian, for example, may have liver-damaging effects. Despite this, I will often recommend natural remedies to patients simply because they are natural. In cases where that little "push" is needed, they may be helpful. I am also not convinced that the data linking these substances to bodily harm is as bad as the data regarding the use of some prescription sleep aids.

MELATONIN

Melatonin is a hormone our brain makes naturally when darkness sets in. Initially, melatonin was obtained from cows or pigs, and in the early days it was packaged as a natural supplement. Today melatonin is synthesized in the lab and is available in any pharmacy. It's what I usually recommend as a starter, particularly if I don't feel a prescription medication is necessary. I prefer to see if we can do things naturally and then, if need be, I'll follow up with something stronger.

In its pill or liquid form, melatonin can aid in helping us get to sleep as well as help keeping us asleep, and it can be used on an as-needed basis. I usually start patients on 1 mg to 3 mg of melatonin, either thirty minutes before sleep, if they are having trouble initiating sleep, or right at bedtime if they wake during the night. The pill or liquid form can be found at virtually any supermarket or pharmacy.

Melatonin is typically safe,[1] but, like anything, there may be side effects. Some patients require as much as 10 mg, but this may lead to feeling hungover the next day and may be masking OSA or other real problems. In cases where people stop taking melatonin, it is usually either because it did not work well enough or it gave them nightmares. Additionally, there are suggestions that melatonin can affect fertility, but this is not definitive.

Another interesting fact about melatonin is that it's one of the most powerful antioxidants in the body. Antioxidants help our bodies fight illnesses that result from oxygen free radicals, which are the by-products of metabolism and other reactions that occur naturally in our body. As we will discuss in chapter 11, reduced production of melatonin is one of the theories as to why people who work overnight shifts for many years are at a higher risk of developing cancer.

VALERIAN

Valerian is a flowering plant native to Europe and parts of Asia. Its name comes from the Latin *valere*, "to be strong and healthy." Valerian has been used as a medicinal herb since at least the time of ancient Greece and Rome. The famous physician Hippocrates described its properties, and Galen later prescribed it as a remedy for insomnia.

Throughout history, it has been used as a sedative, antiseptic, anticonvulsant, and migraine treatment. It has even been administered for relief of menstrual pain, since it has antispasm properties.

Valerian is thought to enhance the properties of one of the main sedating substances in the brain and central nervous system, gamma-aminobutyric acid (GABA). There are different preparations, including valerian itself and a valerian-hops combination. Taking it thirty to sixty minutes before bed can be effective as an as-needed treatment, but some reports[2] say that it can take a couple weeks for it to take effect. A reasonable dose to try is 300 mg to 450 mg.

Larger doses of valerian may result in stomach pain; apathy; and a feeling of mental dullness or mild depression, dizziness, or drowsiness. As with any sleep aid, these potential side effects should be considered before driving or operating heavy or hazardous equipment. Abnormally high doses of valerian at night have been associated with a hangover-like effect the next morning.

Because valerian can produce central nervous system depression, it should not be used if you are drinking alcohol or taking benzodiazepines, barbiturates, opiates, kava, or antihistamine drugs. Additionally, as mentioned, some data[3] suggest that valerian may harm the liver over the short term (i.e., a few days to several months) if it is taken in combination with scutellaria (commonly called skullcap). Withdrawal symptoms following long-term use have also been reported. As with any of these substances, a discussion with a doctor is the right way to go before taking them.

CHERRY EXTRACT

Cherry juice is a natural source of melatonin and the amino acid tryptophan. Tryptophan is the building block of melatonin, which we talked about at the start, and serotonin, which many people know is linked to depression. Many antidepressants work by increasing the amount of serotonin in the brain. The ruby red pigments in tart cherry juice contain an enzyme that reduces inflammation in the body and decreases the breakdown of tryptophan, allowing it to work longer in the body.

CHAMOMILE

Derived from the Greek term for "Earth apple," chamomile is the name for several daisy-like plants used in herb infusions for medicinal purposes. Chamomile preparations are used to treat conditions as disparate as hay fever, inflammation, muscle spasm, menstrual disorders, ulcers, gastrointestinal disorder, hemorrhoids, and insomnia.

When used for sleep, the chemical compounds within chamomile are thought to interact with GABA (just like valerian), giving it the relaxing properties that can be helpful for sleep.

A substance found in chamomile tea known as apigenin may interact with medications, potentially causing harm. Drug interactions can be seen with antiplatelet agents, anticoagulant agents, non-steroidal anti-inflammatory agents (i.e., acetaminophen), and possibly with antiarrhythmic and antihypertensive agents.

Because chamomile has been shown to cause uterine contractions that can lead to miscarriage, the National Institutes of Health (NIH) recommends that pregnant and nursing mothers think twice when considering its use. Again, always check with a doctor before taking chamomile.

OTHER POSSIBILITIES WORTH TRYING

Magnesium has been shown to help relax the central nervous system, which is why it is thought to help sleep. It is present in green leafy vegetables, wheat germ, pumpkin seeds, and almonds. Magnesium can interact with many different medications. Too much can cause serious cardiac issues, so always consult a physician before starting it.

One natural insomnia remedy that has stood the test of time is sipping warm milk before bed. The best sleep-inducing foods include a combination of protein and carbohydrates. It is commonly thought that the reason we feel sleepy after a big Thanksgiving dinner is due to the large amount of tryptophan in turkey meat. In all likelihood, it is because we eat a large load of carbohydrates along with the turkey, which produces what is called postprandial somnolence, otherwise known as a "food coma."

Lavender oil has been a folk remedy for many years in many cultures, and using it with a warm bath before bed can help to calm things down and induce sleep.

L-theanine is a substance found in green tea leaves, and some believe it can reduce heart rate and immune responses to stress. It's thought to work for insomnia by its anxiety-reduction properties. Again, please talk to a doctor before using it.

Some of the teas on the market also work well for some people. Sleepytime Tea, which is made from herbs and other botanicals, is one that claims to aid relaxation and promote sleep.

Finally, while we're on the subject of food and drink, remember that it is not a good idea to go to bed with a full stomach. Nor is it ideal to go to bed starving. One simple thing to try is having a light snack thirty minutes before bed, such as half a banana with a tablespoon of peanut butter or a whole-wheat cracker with some cheese.

SUMMARY AND ACTION PLAN

There are many herbal and natural substances out there that can be used in the treatment of insomnia. However, the data are not very exhaustive, and there are many conflicting and seemingly contradictory reports about the use and safety of these substances. As with all things in this book, you definitely need to let your doctor know what you have tried and what you are currently taking, prescription or otherwise.

- Start with the simple stuff—warm milk before bed, lavender oil, a light snack, and so on may work.
- Good sleep habits are a must—if you need a refresher, turn back to chapters 1 and 4 and read up on sleep hygiene and meditation.
- The first natural substance I have my patients try is melatonin—it is considered safe, and may be effective for you.
- Other substances, like valerian or magnesium, may work, but you should check with your doctor before taking.

6

OBSTRUCTIVE SLEEP APNEA

Obstructive sleep apnea is a serious condition. It does its damage over the years, and it can result in strokes, heart attacks, and other major problems.

The term *apnea* refers to a temporary stoppage of breathing. Obstructive sleep apnea, or OSA, is the most common form of breathing problems in sleep and is thought to affect 20–30 percent of men and 10–15 percent of women in North America.[1] As society ages and gets heavier, OSA is almost certainly going to become even more prevalent.

When we are awake, the brain signals the upper airway to stay open; this includes the tongue, the tonsils, the uvula (the "punching bag" in the back of the throat), and the soft palate (the back part of the "roof" of the mouth). When we fall asleep, our muscles relax, which makes the upper airway smaller.

When someone is suffering with OSA, it means his or her airway has not just become smaller, but that it actually closes off many times throughout the night. Usually, the tongue falls toward the back of the throat, which triggers the brain to either fully wake itself up or go into a state of very light sleep. As a result, someone with OSA may be sleeping a full eight hours, but because the person's airway is repeatedly closing off through the night, the quality of the sleep may be so impaired that the person wakes up totally unrefreshed.

For one or two nights, OSA is not a major problem. Over the years, however, serious cases of OSA have effects on blood pressure, blood sugar, and body weight. Additionally, many people with OSA complain of grinding their teeth. They may have morning headaches. There can even be complaints of tinnitus (ringing in the ears). Some complain of needing to wake up to urinate throughout the night (which in many cases is falsely blamed on prostate issues), and there can be gastric reflux symptoms (like heartburn).

When someone has unobstructed breathing, the airway is totally wide open. There is plenty of space in the nasal passages, as well as in the area behind the tongue, and air that is breathed in and out can move without causing any commotion.

In the case of snoring, the air passages are a little "tight." This can occur as a result of a number of issues: blocked nasal passages (which is often caused by a cold or allergies); the tongue and soft tissue falling to the back of the throat; excess weight; being dehydrated; having alcohol or certain medications in the body; exposure to smoking; or, as in the case of children especially, large tonsils. As inhaled air rushes by a tightened airway, it becomes very turbulent and causes the soft tissues to vibrate quickly—which results in the sounds of snoring.

If the airway closes off completely—either from the soft palate, the tongue, or a combination falling to the back of the throat—we have an apnea, which is a stoppage of breathing. By definition, an apnea lasts at least ten seconds, but it can be as long as a minute or more. An apnea may then trigger the brain to make the sufferer wake up, move, gasp for air, or do something else to improve the situation. Again, this is not harmful if it happens once or twice—but after years and years of experiencing it nightly, we could have a problem.

Diagrams of these three scenarios—normal breathing, snoring, and OSA—can be found online by doing a Google image search for "obstructive sleep apnea."

Like insomnia, OSA becomes more frequent as we get older, and this is true for both men and women. Premenopausal women are actually protected against OSA, and while this means they can certainly still have it, the likelihood is less. Once estrogen and progesterone are no longer produced, which is what happens during menopause, the risk in women almost reaches the level of men.

Estrogen is responsible for the deposition of fat cells that make women look different from men. When it is no longer available, fat tissue may become deposited in areas that normally would not have had any, in particular the neck area. With more fat tissue deposited around the neck area (microscopically, mind you), the airway is essentially smaller, and that can increase the risk of OSA.

Progesterone also has many effects on the body, including its role as a respiratory stimulant. Without it, a postmenopausal woman may not be breathing deeply in sleep, which can increase the risk of OSA.

The way we characterize OSA is by how often the airway closes each hour over the course of a night's sleep. Less than five events per hour is normal. If you took one thousand people at random and had them do a sleep test, the majority would have two or three events per hour, and this is fine. Mild OSA consists of five to fifteen stoppages of breathing per hour, moderate OSA is fifteen to thirty stoppages per hour, and severe OSA is more than thirty stoppages per hour.

People who have mild and perhaps moderate OSA for a period of time are not usually affected in a major way healthwise, but people suffering with the severe form are at risk for other health concerns. After ten or fifteen years, OSA can have a big impact on mortality. We're talking cardiovascular illness, strokes, heart attacks, and blood sugar problems. Even cancer has been linked to severe OSA. It's a serious condition because it can take years off a person's life.

What can we do about it? One answer is the mask and hose device that we mentioned earlier. It is usually referred to by its initials, CPAP, which stands for continuous positive airway pressure, and it is worn when asleep. CPAP involves sending pressurized air through the nasal passages alone, or through the nasal passages and mouth, down to the back of the throat. It prevents the tongue and the soft tissues from falling down and clogging the airway. Basically, CPAP acts as an airway splint to keep the air passages open throughout the night. It does not actually breathe for the user; rather, it clears the air passages so that snoring and, more importantly, OSA do not occur.

There are different types of CPAPs, and people who use them often have different experiences. While there are many "horror" stories about CPAP, others find them easy to adapt to. One of my patients, Chris, has been using a CPAP for years. He has an interesting history.

> I'm fifty-seven. I first realized I had a sleep problem approximately twenty years ago. My ex-girlfriend was sleeping over at the time, and she said, wow, you are a loud snorer. It wasn't happening all the time, and I had no idea I was snoring, but when I did it was obviously annoying and was keeping her awake. I didn't do anything about it

for a while. Then a year or so later I was out camping with friends. We were in different tents, and the next morning my buddies all got together and said, wow, you are a loud snorer.

That did it for me. I went to an ear, nose, and throat (ENT) doctor at that point and he gave me an exam. He said I had a very large uvula, which he described as a piece of skin tissue that dangles at the back of my throat. He said that might be the problem. He gave me a home sleep-study test that consisted of a piece of tubing that went from my nose to a recording device. I slept with it overnight and sent it back to him. Next time I saw him he said, yes, you are a heavy snorer, and it might help if we shave your uvula. I said, okay, and went in for surgery. It was an office procedure that took maybe ten minutes. I had a sore throat for a week, but I took the test again a few weeks later and the snoring seemed better.

It actually improved for a while, but then the problem came back. I had put on weight during this period, and someone suggested that might be the problem. Whatever. One day I was talking to a friend who plays bass in my band, and he said his doctor thinks he has apnea and he's going in for a sleep-study test. That sounded like a good idea. I went to a sleep center, and they hooked me up with electrodes and discovered I had apnea and it was waking me up during the night.

The episodes were very mild, and when the technician gave me a continuous positive airway pressure (CPAP) machine, she said the pressure was set very low, sort of what they do for kids. That made me feel good, and it wasn't all that bad. But the CPAP came with a nasal mask, and at times I felt my mouth opening and I realized I was still breathing through my mouth. Sometimes when I was watching TV, I'd fall asleep, and I'd wake and hear myself snoring. It wasn't severe, but I was still having episodes where I stopped breathing.

I went back to the sleep doctor, got retested, and was given a new machine with a full-face mask. I've been using it ever since. I don't snore when I have the machine on, and I get a good night's sleep with it. I've lost some weight, and that's probably helped too.

I take the CPAP machine with me on vacations. It's been to the Bahamas, Holland, and Paris. I just have to leave a little extra space in my suitcase. I had to get an adaptor for the current in Europe, but that was easy. I don't think I've missed more than one or two night's sleep in the last ten years.

Some thoughts on Chris's experience:

- People who have obstructive sleep apnea often learn about it from a friend: "My friend/girlfriend/bed partner tells me I am a loud snorer," is how conversations with a new patient often begin. Hopefully, with increased public awareness, people will be more willing to undergo testing. Not all snoring is OSA, and not all OSA necessarily has snoring as a feature—but it's a good starting point.

- The surgery Chris went through is called an uvulectomy. It can be combined with a shaving down of the soft palate, and the combination is called—sorry, but here goes—an uvulopalatopharyngoplasty, mercifully known by the initials UPPP. It has fallen out of favor during the past few years, largely because it may not be fully effective for OSA. It can reduce snoring, but remember, a major reason for OSA has to do with the tongue falling to the back of the throat, and this type of surgery would not help with that.

- There is a difference between home testing and in-lab testing. Home testing is a viable option if the problem appears to be OSA. Compared to an in-lab polysomnogram (PSG), which consists of many electrodes monitoring an assortment of different parameters, a home sleep test simply measures airflow (via a sensor in the nose/mouth) and oxygen levels (an oximeter on the finger). Although most people tend to find a home test easier to tolerate and more comfortable than an in-lab PSG, the problem is that home tests do not measure actual sleep time or account for other problems that may occur during sleep. But for simple OSA, a home test is usually fine.

- Having OSA can make it difficult to lose weight. Once OSA is treated, it may realign the hormones that control hunger, and it may raise energy levels and lead to an increased desire/ability to exercise. Both of these would potentially bring about weight loss.

- When a patient really takes to a CPAP, it can be a life changer, and the fact that Chris has no trouble traveling with it speaks volumes. While there are portable CPAP units, the base unit of the standard device is small enough in most cases for travel. I often tell patients to remove the humidification unit when they travel. This reduces the size of the machine and, since humidification is not necessary for the CPAP to work, the patient may only be losing out on a bit of comfort and nothing else.

- There are three main types of CPAP interfaces: the full-face mask (which covers nose and mouth), the nasal mask (covering just the nose), and nasal pillows ("plugs" that sit in the nostrils themselves). The choice of mask is based on several factors: comfort and size are the big ones, but if a patient is strictly a mouth breather with a constantly stuffed nose, a nasal interface may not be effective. In those cases, we will opt for a full-face mask. I personally try to avoid the full-face masks if possible, because they are bulkier. In the right patient—someone like Chris—they can be incredibly helpful.

- The "classic" version of testing for, and treating, OSA is done with an overnight sleep test followed by an overnight CPAP test on another night to figure out what settings and equipment the person will need. Another option that is sometimes favored by patients, called a split-night test, encompasses both the diagnostic and the treatment arms of OSA. The advantage is that it takes place over one night (as opposed to two) and is usually informative enough to get the person on CPAP faster. The downside is that it is one night, and sufficient information may not be garnered from the test.

Another patient, Arthur, had a slightly different but equally positive experience with CPAP.

> I'm sixty-nine, and my sleep problems started twenty or so years ago. I was around fifty at the time. I ran the public relations and advertising department for a global Wall Street investment bank. It was a typical Type A executive's life during an extremely stressful time.
>
> Over the years, I had been given more and more responsibilities; worked longer, harder hours; and exercised significantly less than I had in my younger days. I entertained guests a couple of nights a week at dinner and four or five days a week at lunch. It was easy to find comfort in food, and I discovered I was a stress eater. The pounds snuck up on me and I became extremely overweight.
>
> I also found I wanted to take naps after lunch and often felt overwhelmingly fatigued at the end of the day. I mentioned this to my internist at my annual physical, and after four or five years he suggested that I go to a sleep clinic. I followed up and spent a night with wires attached to all different parts of my body. I left at about 5:30 in the morning, having been told I had gone through the proper

number of sleep cycles. I got the diagnosis a few days later of moderate sleep apnea.

When the sleep doctor heard from the clinic, he urged me to get a CPAP, which, he told me, consisted of a mask and tubes that drove air into my nose and kept the airway open. It gave me a semblance of better sleep for a while, but at a high cost. In addition to being uncomfortable, the equipment rubbed hair off my head and I lost a quarter of an inch of hair on my eyebrows. The mask was also awkward to use. It was difficult to get the right settings and to get it to fit right.

My next stop was the Weill Cornell Center for Sleep Medicine, where I spent a night in the sleep clinic. The results were different this time, but it was now years later and by this point I was a very different person. I had undergone triple-bypass heart surgery five years earlier. After the operation, I left my job; started working out in the gym almost every day; went on a strict, very healthy diet; and lost a significant amount of weight.

Although the test showed I had gone from a moderate to a very mild form of sleep apnea, Dr. Barone said I probably would never be fully cured. He brought me up to speed on the ergonomics of the new CPAP equipment. I spent another night in the sleep clinic, trying out several options and settling on a new mask. There were a number of issues involving the fit and the equipment took some getting used to, but the adjustment period was short and it was worth the relief of getting a good night's sleep and waking up feeling refreshed.

Many aspects of my life have improved, the most important being the delight and joy that a night's sleep brings. I wear the mask every night now, and it works. I go to sleep around 11 p.m. and get up at 7:30 or 8. I wake up occasionally for an age-appropriate trip to the bathroom. I have an occasional period of sleeplessness during the night when I'll wake up for a half hour or so, but I stay in bed and get back to sleep.

The combination of weight loss, diet, exercise, and the new mask has not made a new man of me but certainly a better one. My wife and I traveled recently for a wedding, and the CPAP equipment rode along with us. It's a little kit and it's easy to pack. It travels well and works perfectly in Paris and other places we've been.

Two final thoughts. First, my father was never diagnosed as such, but I did some research and found that it is highly likely that he too had sleep apnea. Second, I was a little disappointed that my significant weight loss and new fitness program hadn't cured me of sleep apnea. But I understand that the body changes as you grow older, which is when sleep apnea often begins. I'm extremely happy with my health at this point. My sleeping health is quite good, and I've got to believe the new CPAP equipment has added many enjoyable years to my life.

Arthur's experience gives us a lot to think about:

- For starters, stress often leads to an unhealthy balance, which can then be followed by negative consequences: weight gain, poor sleep, and an overall sense of a lack of well-being. Additionally, as we know, a lack of physical exercise can affect our ability to sleep well. We are designed to move. When we don't, it's as if our body has not "burned off" the excess energy, and it's difficult to fall asleep at night. Multiple studies have shown that simply adding twenty to thirty minutes of regular exercise a day can have a profound effect on insomnia.
- We all normally have an after-lunch feeling of tiredness. Technically, it is called postprandial somnolence. Our circadian signal (which keeps us awake) normally dips in the early afternoon, which is probably why people in other countries have siestas. With the typical American diet (excess carbs, not enough vegetables), this signal can be magnified. Add it to the kind of sleep disorder that Arthur has, and it explains his feelings of fatigue.
- People who try CPAP for the first time often have the same complaint: it's uncomfortable, causes claustrophobia, and is noisy, all of which are completely valid. Sometimes it takes extra effort on the part of the doctor—as well as the home care medical company that supplies the actual equipment—to work with the patient to get the right mask. In some cases I will prescribe a short course of a sleeping pill like zolpidem (Ambien) or have patients try melatonin for a couple weeks as they adjust to life with the CPAP. This can get them "over the hump" and increase satisfaction with CPAP in time.
- Even in those who are very thin, OSA can still be present. It is important to note that the anatomy/physiology of the upper airway in someone with OSA tends to be "tight," which can set them up for airway closures in sleep. In some OSA patients, this has little

to do with weight, and is rather based on age and genetics, as Arthur's case points out.

- The key takeaway from Arthur's history is that even if someone tried CPAP in the past but couldn't tolerate it or didn't want to continue, that is not to say we can't make it work in the future. In this day and age, with the field moving ahead rapidly, new masks and equipment are being designed and refined regularly. It can absolutely be worth a retry by those who have been initially disappointed.
- Nowadays it is very rare for the travel/airport authorities to have an issue with someone bringing a CPAP on board. In isolated cases, where my patients are traveling to less-technologically advanced countries, I will write a letter on their behalf explaining what the CPAP is and why they should be allowed to bring it with them. It usually does the trick.

A common question I get is whether the CPAP is "breathing" for the patient. The answer is no. The CPAP machine is blowing a continuous stream of pressurized air, but it is not a ventilator like someone in an intensive care unit would be on. In fact, CPAP allows patients to breathe on their own, without the airway blockages of OSA occurring. If CPAP is stopped for a night, the OSA may go back to where it was before but certainly not get worse. Some people think they will become "addicted" or habituated to the CPAP, which is not correct.

There are different kinds of masks, and new types are coming out every year or so. If you talk to people who tried CPAP twenty years ago, they typically say something like, "I had a huge Darth Vader thing on my face, and it was horrible." These days we have much smaller interfaces.

Another question I frequently get regarding this issue is, "Will my OSA become worse if I use the CPAP and then stop?" The answer is no; it will go back to what it was before treatment.

Chronic snoring and OSA produce inflammation of the upper airway. Inflammation results in swelling of soft tissues (similar to what happens in a sprained ankle), and the airway is further tightened as a result of this swelling. Adding CPAP to the mix reduces the inflammation. As a result, in the case of someone who uses CPAP nightly but then stops for a night, the bed partner may say their partner is not

snoring anymore. While this is correct, it does not mean that the OSA
has been cured. Rather, a few more nights without CPAP will result in
the inflammation returning and the OSA will revert back to where it
started, snoring and all.

The bottom line is that CPAP does work, and there is a large amount
of medical literature showing how effective it is.

That said, not everyone can tolerate CPAP. The second most common treatment for OSA is known as a mandibular advancement device
(MAD), which is a mouth guard that fits over the upper and the lower
teeth. When placed in the mouth right before sleep, it moves the lower
jaw (the mandible) forward a few millimeters. By moving the jaw forward, the tongue and the soft tissues are moved away from the back of
the throat, reducing the likelihood of obstructions occurring during
sleep. This is good for mild to moderate cases of OSA, but it also can be
useful in severe cases of OSA for someone who can't tolerate CPAP.

A high-quality mandibular advancement device is made by a special-
ly trained dentist, and it can be expensive, ranging from $500 to $2,500.
A "boil and bite" version is much less expensive ($50–$100), but not as
effective and not as durable. If someone just snores without actually
having OSA (as determined from a sleep test), I may start by recom-
mending nasal strips, which are narrow bandage-like strips that fit over
the outside of the nose and help open the nasal passages. I also may
recommend a "boil and bite" MAD from an online source. I would not
typically recommend either for someone who has an actual case of
OSA.

A good example of how a MAD can fit into the treatment picture of
OSA can be seen with another patient of mine, Michael.

I'm about to turn fifty-nine, and my first memory of sleep problems
goes back to the mid-1980s when I was starting a new job. I'm sure I
was nervous about the job, but I was already having problems. They
typically took the form of waking up too early. I never had trouble
getting to sleep and staying asleep for part of the night, but I would
wake up at 4 or 5 in the morning.

That was one part of the problem. The other was having the very
distinct feeling of never having a restful night's sleep or never having
sleep that was rejuvenating. I might sleep but I'd wake up feeling
extremely tired.

I recall trying to deal with the problem with my internist, who gave me medication to help me sleep. I don't remember what it was, but it wasn't particularly helpful. A few years later I went to a sleep doctor who recommended an overnight study in a sleep center. When it was done, he concluded I didn't have significant sleep apnea, and he put me on a different medication and suggested tutoring in behavioral modification.

The sleep doctor also recommended a mouth device for snoring. He said it was called a mandibular advancement device (MAD) and it resembles something a boxer wears when he's in the ring. It makes your lower jaw jut forward, which opens up the air passage. It helped reduce my snoring for a while, but I was still making life miserable for my wife. She's a light sleeper and I'm a poor sleeper, and that's a very bad combination. I would snore, kick my legs, and flop around during the night.

I first saw Dr. Barone three or four years ago, and his initial approach was to work on sleep hygiene and behavioral things, and attempt to modify and lessen my medications. I had been on a cocktail of sleep medications, and we tried to cut it back. Ultimately he decided to put me through another sleep study, and that revealed that I had sleep apnea when I was lying on my back.

The behavioral things I now try to do involve a little meditation, sleeping in a cool bedroom with all the lights off, and no TV or computers close to bedtime. It all works if I'm conscientious about doing it.

Dr. Barone tried to get me to go the CPAP route at one point, but I could never get used to it. So he would move on to something else. He'd say something like, "This is not going to be a cure-all, but maybe we ought to try making the mouth device a little more aggressive." That meant adjusting the MAD so my jaw jutted forward a little more than it had been. It took a little getting used to and my jaw doesn't immediately snap back to its normal position when I get up in the morning, but it usually does within ten minutes or so, and I think the more aggressive setting helps.

At one point I lost some weight and that helped too. These days I occasionally do the behavioral stuff. I use the mouth device, and I take eszopiclone (Lunesta) and doxepin. I also take lorazepam, which is an antianxiety drug that relaxes you and makes you sleepy. We're in the process of adjusting the medications, but this group seems to be working.

Before I tried the CPAP, I tried another device at Dr. Barone's suggestion, something that had inflated balloons in the back. It was supposed to keep you from sleeping on your back. It didn't really work but, at Dr. Barone's suggestion, I moved on to a backpack that contains a beach ball, and that seems to work.

Here's the thing: We're both open to trying different things, and it's been very helpful. I'm sleeping better and waking up feeling more rested. I see Dr. Barone every four months or so, and I'm much happier than I was three or four years ago.

Some things to consider from Michael's case:

- An overnight sleep test can often be of great benefit when we are looking for things that may wake someone up. Michael and I decided to hold off on a repeat sleep test initially because his prior one was benign. However, as people age and in some cases gain weight, the possibility of OSA goes up. I was glad in a way that we found his OSA because it was something I knew we could improve upon.
- The adverse effects of a MAD can be jaw pain, excess salivation, or temporary bite changes. Like CPAP, a MAD may be uncomfortable for some people, but for those who can tolerate it, a MAD can be a nice alternative. As in Michael's case, a dentist may have to fine-tune it to accomplish opening the airway.

In cases in which medications are needed, I always try to make sure that all potential problems are addressed as best we can. In Michael's case, it was important to make sure his OSA was addressed with the MAD before prescribing eszopiclone (Lunesta) or lorazepam (Ativan). These medications can worsen OSA on a night-to-night basis by relaxing the upper airway tissues further, leading to more obstructions to breathing. Alcohol can do the same thing, and we often also see it when we use benzodiazepine (alprazolam [Xanax], clonazepam [Klonopin], lorazepam [Ativan], etc.) and the non-benzodiazepine (zolpidem [Ambien], eszopiclone [Lunesta], etc.) medications that we discussed in chapter 4.

Positional therapy is another option for dealing with OSA. Sometimes, people with OSA have breathing blockages only when on their back—this is known as positional OSA. In these people, stoppages of breathing happen because gravity pulls the soft tissues and tongue down toward the back of the throat, which closes up the airway, when they fall asleep. Many times, the bed partners of my patients with positional OSA will say something like, "I elbow him, he rolls over, and then he's fine." With this background, let's take a look at Patrick's case:

I'm sixty-three, and I've had sleep problems for a long time. I used to wake up in the middle of the night, panting and feeling like I was out of breath. It was scary and very strange. I was in my forties then. I didn't do anything about it at the time, and for some reason it got better.

Then, maybe three or four years ago, the problem came back. My wife, who is the one who noticed it, told me I was snoring on and off a good part of the night.

In July of 2015, I spent a night at the sleep center at the Weill Cornell Center for Sleep Medicine. It wasn't the most fun thing I've ever done, but it was pleasant enough. You have your own room and your own bathroom. They hooked me up with electrodes on my temples and nose to keep track of what was happening while I slept, and they put a cuff on my arm to measure my blood pressure. It was a little uncomfortable but nothing really bad. According to the people at the center, I slept about seven hours, right through the night.

Dr. Barone reviewed the data the next day and found that my problem comes when I sleep on my back. In addition to snoring, he found I had sleep apnea whenever I was flat on my back. To deal with it, he gave me a belt that comes with inflatable balloons that he said to wear when I went to sleep. It's like a weight-lifting belt, but it's made out of Velcro. You inflate the balloons and slip them into the belt, which you put across your chest with the balloons in the back. The idea is that when you roll over onto your back, it's uncomfortable so you turn onto your side.

I haven't gotten into the habit of using it all the time, probably because I don't have trouble falling asleep most nights. Sometimes I'm so tired I just get in bed and the next thing I know I'm out.

At this point I use the Velcro belt three or four nights a week. When I do, it seems to do the trick. I never get up in the middle of the night gasping for air any more, but on the days I forget to use the belt, my wife says I snore like crazy.

The symptoms Patrick reports can be quite typical of a person suffering with positional OSA. Some other thoughts on his case:

- What is interesting is that Patrick reports the symptoms improved over time. Usually, OSA in all forms tends to get worse as we age. Sometimes people with OSA have no idea they are suffering with it. So it may be that Patrick was spending less time on his back during that period, he lost some weight, or a combination of the two. The point I am trying to make is that chances are the OSA didn't just "go away."

- Similar to our other patients, Patrick's reservations about a sleep test are common, but they tend to be short-lived once the initial shock of being wired up wears off. Often, patients will have no idea if they even slept at all with all the electrodes taped to them. But fortunately, with the technology we use, we can see from the brain waves whether someone is asleep or awake, and it is during the time they spend asleep that we are able to find out if they have *obstructive* sleep apnea. I always tell my patients to not worry about how much they will sleep during the test, because any time they do sleep will help us to determine if OSA is there or not.

- Patrick had moderate OSA throughout the night, but when he was on his back, it became much worse. I suggested he try CPAP, but he understandably did not want to at first. For this reason, I provided the positional belt to keep him off his back.

- A positional belt can be very effective for this type of OSA. Unfortunately, as Patrick points out, it may be uncomfortable and patients may neglect to use it.

- I am hoping I can convince Patrick to use the belt more often. Every night would be ideal. If that doesn't happen, I have told him we will have to at least try CPAP. Like many cases, Patrick's is an ongoing process and we will work together to come up with the best solution.

Let's finish this chapter with a look at some of the other things that can be done to help improve OSA.

Alcohol and smoking are two things known to worsen snoring and OSA. Reducing or eliminating these substances can improve both snoring and OSA, at least to some degree. Alcohol helps us relax, but it also relaxes the upper airway muscles. When the tongue and soft tissues in the upper airway relax, that can lead to turbulent airflow. This can cause quick vibrations, which result in snoring. Some people say they only snore when they drink, and this is why.

I strongly advise my patients with OSA, particularly those who refuse or cannot tolerate treatment, to either avoid alcohol altogether or reduce consumption and to keep at least a few hours from the time of their last drink to the time they go to bed.

Smoking has many well-reported adverse health effects. But what is not well known is that it can worsen OSA by irritating the upper airway. The swelling that results from inflammation is best seen by looking at what happens with a sprained ankle: the ankle swells up and it may be difficult to put on a shoe. In the upper airway, when there is swelling from tobacco smoke, the space through which inhaled air passes becomes smaller. As we now know, a smaller airway results in snoring and OSA.

Weight loss can also be very helpful when dealing with OSA. Not surprisingly, having excess weight around the neck will make the diameter of the airway smaller. Not everyone who has OSA is overweight, but for those who are, losing weight can be a great first step to reducing the problem.

These treatments are all very conservative ways to improve snoring and OSA. But what about more advanced technologies or techniques?

A new treatment called hypoglossal nerve stimulation recently arrived on the scene. This is a procedure done by an ear, nose, and throat (ENT) surgeon, who implants a device, not unlike a pacemaker, into the right chest wall. Several brands use this technology, all of which share at least one commonality—a wire in the neck (under the skin) which is attached to the nerve that controls the tongue. This special nerve is called the hypoglossal nerve.

Once the stimulator is implanted and calibrated, the patient sets it remotely at bedtime. When activated, it stiffens the tongue muscle. While this sounds like science fiction, it means that the possibility of the tongue falling backward and closing off the airway becomes much smaller. Since this is relatively new, we tend to reserve hypoglossal nerve stimulation for cases where someone has severe OSA and can't tolerate any other treatment. In the future, however, it may be much more commonly used.

There are two other less well-known treatments for OSA. I will mention them only briefly, because they don't tend to be used much these days. The Winx system is a machine like CPAP. Unlike CPAP, which forces air down the throat, the Winx system works by "sucking" the soft tissue of the upper airway forward while it stabilizes the tongue, making the upper airway space larger. The Winx system has several problems, including the fact that insurance carriers do not usually cover it. Another problem is that there is no way of knowing beforehand whether it will work. I have a very few patients using the Winx system at the time of this writing, but those who are on it tend to like it and tolerate it well.

Provent, another relatively new treatment, uses what is called micro-valve technology to keep the airway open. The actual device consists of two adhesive patches that are worn over the nostrils during sleep. These patches work by allowing the patient to breathe in freely; upon breathing out, the valve closes and air passing through the nose is directed toward the back of the throat, opening the airway until the start of the next breath. Provent has not worked well for the patients I have tried it on, and the medical literature[2] is not encouraging.

The last thing I want to mention here regarding treatment for OSA has to do with the tonsils and adenoids. The tonsils are two balls of tissue in the back of the throat that, when inflamed, can swell up and make the airway small. Adenoids, unlike tonsils, cannot be seen without special equipment, as they lie inside the upper airway. Both of these are especially important in children when we talk about snoring and OSA.

Between the ages of two and eight, tonsils are largest compared to the size of the rest of the airway. If a child is snoring at night, sleepy during the day, or hyperactive (children may behave similarly to those with attention-deficit hyperactivity disorder when they are sleep deprived), it makes sense to discuss it with a doctor. Children can actually have OSA, and a sleep test would be diagnostic. In that case, if the tonsils are large, the plan would most likely be to remove them, along with the adenoids.

Removing the tonsils and adenoids (or sometimes just either) can have a tremendous impact on the life of a child suffering with OSA. Removing them in adults comes with risk, and while the procedure may improve snoring, it would not necessarily have a huge impact on OSA.

As we close this chapter, I want to take another look at the difference between obstructive sleep apnea and central sleep apnea. Obstructive sleep apnea is a condition where the patient can't breathe normally because of an obstruction in the upper airway; we talked about these obstructions to breathing throughout this chapter. In central sleep apnea, which we discuss in the next chapter, the brain doesn't send proper signals to the muscles that control breathing. This results in pauses of breathing where the person doesn't even seem to be trying. It sounds scary, but hopefully I can shed some light on it for you and your loved ones.

SUMMARY AND ACTION PLAN

Snoring is a very common condition in which vibratory sounds occur when the upper airway is partially blocked off. Obstructive sleep apnea (OSA) is a common disorder in which there are repetitive stoppages of breathing while someone is asleep, usually due to the tongue and/or soft tissues falling toward the back of the throat. Snoring can be seen in cases of OSA, but not all with OSA snore, and vice versa.

In dealing with snoring and OSA, the place to start is by reviewing your own sleep experiences and discussing them with your bed partner.

- Make a list of how often you wake up in the middle of the night and what you think it is that wakes you up—a snort, a gasp for air, a feeling like you can't breathe, sweating, or a feeling of panic from repeated dreams of drowning, being choked, or whatever.
- Ask your bed partner if you snore (if he or she hasn't already told you), if you stop breathing during the night, or if you gasp or sound like you are choking in your sleep.
- A bed partner's report can be very helpful, but it isn't everything. If you wake up multiple times through the night (even just to go to the bathroom) and/or wake in the morning feeling unrefreshed, these would be good reasons to have a conversation with a sleep doctor. There are many reasons for both of these situations— prostate problems, for example, which cause men to wake fre-quently—but it can't hurt to have that discussion.
- An overnight sleep test can determine if you have simple snoring or actual OSA.
- Depending on the level of severity of OSA, multiple treatments are available:

- continuous positive airway pressure (CPAP)
- mandibular advancement device (MAD)
- Winx
- Provent
- ENT surgery
- hypoglossal nerve stimulation

Other steps to take:

- If you are overweight, losing weight should help with both snoring and OSA.
- Sleeping on your side in the fetal position is the best way to sleep, for both your airway's sake as well as your neck and lower back.
- Reducing alcohol, stopping smoking, and staying hydrated through the day can help.
- Treating snoring with nasal strips (Breathe Right is a brand many people like), nasal dilators (little plastic cones that fit in the nostrils), or a nasal patch (brand name Theravent) can be effective, but they won't be helpful in treating actual OSA.

7

OTHER BREATHING PROBLEMS IN SLEEP

Central sleep apnea (CSA) is similar to obstructive sleep apnea (OSA) in some respects, very different in others. OSA occurs when there is an obstruction in the upper airway, typically caused by the tongue falling back toward the back of the throat. In CSA, the airway is wide open—in fact, another name for it is clear airway apnea. The *central* part of central sleep apnea refers to the fact that the stoppage of breathing is caused by a problem in the *central* nervous system, and is not due to a physical blockage.

In CSA, while patients will often say they don't get the quality sleep they need, their bed partners may not hear the loud snoring and chok-ing noises that tend to be part of OSA. In fact, bed partners will often say the person completely stops trying to breathe, to the point where they make no noise.

As Lisa and Mark learned, the symptoms of CSA can be dramatic and scary to experience.

> My husband, Mark, is in his eighties. He had a triple bypass and a mechanical prosthetic aortic heart valve replacement in the late 1980s. Mark also has progressive congestive heart failure. His cardiac ejection fraction, a measurement of the efficiency of the heart, is less than 25 percent, a very low reading. His condition is further compli-cated by a significant aortic aneurysm.
>
> Three years ago, things were complicated further when Mark became a restless, noisy sleeper. I stopped sleeping and spent my nights observing and listening to him. His breathing was ragged,

horribly noisy, and then he would simply stop breathing, many times per night. Each time I was sure it was the last. Then he would sputter back to irregular breathing and the cycle would start over again.

Mark was unaware of most of this, but he was always tired. We later learned he was having more than eighty incidences of inadequate breathing per hour, and never actually achieved REM sleep. His exhaustion (and mine) became severe. I told his primary care provider that Mark's adult son had been diagnosed with obstructive sleep apnea, and suggested that Mark might have it too.

Mark went in for testing. The doctor discovered he had central sleep apnea, which is not caused by obstruction, a pesky uvula, or snoring, but rather by a brain dysfunction: as he put it, the brain doesn't notify the body to breathe normally. To deal with his type of sleep apnea, Mark would require something called a VPAP device, which, unlike the more common CPAP, is more sophisticated, more intuitive, more expensive, and not fully covered by his insurance.

We were sent to a medical supply therapist who gave us the mask, headgear, hose, reservoir, communication modem, and filters that would become our roommates. In the course of being fitted for the mask, Mark fell asleep. Fast asleep. Comfortably and quietly. From that summer afternoon on, he has not slept a single night without the mask. He has not had a single incident of insomnia or sleep disturbance, and his rate of compliance with the therapy was evaluated in the 99th percentile.

We continued without incident for approximately a year, with his whole medical team agreeing there was a general overall improvement in his well-being. Mark was still very sick, but he had been given a tool for survival that was working. During that year, other medical issues surfaced, but all were resolved with treatment.

Meanwhile, we were living with the VPAP, which is a stern taskmaster. It requires daily cleaning and it drinks only distilled water. Its many parts require regular maintenance and humidity adjustments, and the SD memory card, modem, and other parts require regular replacements. It's daunting. When working optimally, the machine is perfectly silent. But a slip of the mask or a deterioration of the equipment can create leaks, which in turn create noise—a high-pitched whistle that only dogs and wives can hear, or sounds like trumpeter swans flying through the bedroom.

The device takes patience and constant readjustment. Compliance is no easy matter. The machine is always a chief concern, but it is a godsend.

Then, in May of 2015, our world was turned upside down when we got a call from Mark's sleep doctor, who said he had some bad information to share with us. He had just learned about a study being run by ResMed, the manufacturer of Mark's sleep equipment. The study was being ended because of a higher-than-expected incidence of death in a particular study group. As a result, going forward, it appeared that VPAP-based therapy was no longer prudent for patients who had central apnea, congestive heart failure, and an ejection fraction lower than 40 percent—which was precisely Mark's profile.

We were thrown into a tailspin. The only information we could find on the study was limited and uninformative. Mark tried to sleep without the mask and his apnea symptoms instantly returned. It didn't take more than several hours for us to realize he couldn't abandon the therapy. We sought counsel from his other doctors; each one concluded, as we had, that this was something he should continue. His overall prognosis wasn't any better without it, and his quality of life was absolutely improved with it. His cardiologist actually said, "It gave him this year of life." Following that, despite that unsettling phone call and the news about the study, Mark continued to use his equipment every night.

Mark's story gives us a lot to think about. We tend to take our sleep, and our health for that matter, for granted until something goes wrong. For this reason, it is important to learn about healthy sleep and to recognize the signs when things go awry.

- Sleep apnea, be it OSA or CSA, can be very worrisome for bed partners, but it is important for all involved to understand that sufferers do not typically stop breathing to the point that death will occur. What happens is that the body's natural defense mechanisms kick in, leading to a resumption of breathing. While having apnea is certainly dangerous over a period of years, having it for one or two nights will not result in "forgetting to breathe" and death. Over a period of years, however, it can cause strokes, heart attacks, and the like, and they can result in death. It is important to remember this.

- People suffering with sleep apnea (either OSA or CSA) may not necessarily be aware that they have the condition. Like Mark, they often will wake up tired. If a bed partner has the complaints that Lisa describes, it is worth getting checked out, particularly if there is a family history. Mark's history was compelling for sleep apnea, and his finding of severe sleep apnea (more than thirty "events" per hour is considered severe) is not surprising.

- CSA is often seen in the context of congestive heart failure, which is a condition that results from the heart not being able to pump blood effectively. The brain stem, as well as tiny organs in the neck called carotid bodies, have chemical sensors that detect carbon dioxide levels. In cases of congestive heart failure, the sensors are not able to tell that the carbon dioxide levels have changed, simply because blood is not circulating as quickly as it should be. This is a problem because rising carbon dioxide levels are a strong signal to breathe. Thus, the drive to breathe is halted until the carbon dioxide levels rise high enough, and then the person resumes breathing. In cases of CSA, the bed partner may report there is absolutely no effort to breathe during these times, and they are correct. The technical name for this kind of CSA is called Cheyne-Stokes respiration.

- VPAP, which stands for variable positive airway pressure, can "sense" when an intervention is needed. This technology is helpful in cases of CSA in which the body needs a little "push" to breathe again. The most common type of VPAP is called adaptive servo ventilation, or ASV. It is a little different than the continuous positive airway pressure, or CPAP, that we talked about earlier. The CPAP acts as an airway splint, keeping the airway open with a continuous stream of air. VPAP devices provide multiple pressure settings designed to not only keep an airway open (like CPAP), but also to essentially "breathe" for the patient when it senses this is needed. If someone is suffering from an obstructive apnea, the VPAP will raise the pressure to open up the airway; if someone has a central apnea, it will essentially provide a breath to that person, using a backup breathing rate much like a ventilator in a hospital.

- Patients who get over the initial discomfort of VPAP usually find it to be life changing. The more benefit patients feel from a VPAP device, the more inclined they are to continue using it.
- Like anything that interacts with the human body, care must be taken to ensure cleanliness and proper functioning of the VPAP. I urge all my patients to make sure that their supplies (mask, tubing, air filters) are replaced regularly, which typically works out to every three to six months depending on the insurance carrier.
- In cases where the sleep apnea (either OSA or CSA) is severe, I encourage my patients to use the VPAP or CPAP devices every night, as best they can. One night is not going to make a difference, but missing the PAP for two or three nights is not ideal.
- The American Academy of Sleep Medicine has put out a special guideline for patients with CSA and congestive heart failure.[1] If the heart weakness is very severe, the use of a VPAP machine is usually not recommended. However, many doctors feel if there is a benefit to the quality of life, as was true in Mark's case, a lengthy discussion with the patient is absolutely necessary. Ultimately, the decision rests with the patient and doctor, so long as the risks/rewards are clearly evaluated.

Most cases of CSA are called idiopathic, which means there is no specific known reason for it. Other times, we see it in cases of congestive heart failure, as was true with Mark.

Another known cause of CSA is the use of opiates—medications like oxycodone and morphine, for example. Yet another form of CSA occurs when we are at high altitudes, and our body is not adjusted to the elevation. We call this periodic breathing, and it tends to improve once we get used to the high altitude. Finally, there is a form of CSA that presents itself once we treat OSA. This is called "treatment emergent" CSA and can be seen once CPAP has been started.

The way we diagnose CSA is very similar to the way we diagnose OSA in that an overnight sleep test is the key to helping us figure it out. During the overnight sleep test, in cases of OSA, there is repeated effort to breathe, but an obstruction prevents the airflow. In CSA, there's no effort to breathe, and as a result there is no airflow. The reason for the lack of effort is quite complicated, but in simplest terms, the brain and central nervous system simply "forget" to tell the diaphragm to take a breath.

CSA can be just as bad as OSA, so it is important to treat. The prevailing thinking is if someone has one of the underlying conditions associated with CSA, the first step would be to treat the underlying condition. For example, if someone has developed CSA from opiate use, the plan would be to reduce the dosage or switch the patient to another type of medication.

In the case of a weakened heart (congestive heart failure), proper medical management with certain medications may improve the CSA. In cases where improvement does not happen—or if the CSA is idiopathic or the central apneas occur when CPAP has been applied—VPAP may be indicated. The American Academy of Sleep Medicine guideline discussed previously is important to remember. Oxygen therapy or medications are occasionally used to treat CSA, but these have not been as well studied as VPAP.

Like OSA, CSA is a condition that is important to treat, and if there is even a possibility of having it, I always suggest getting tested.

To end this admittedly complicated topic, I would like to mention some of the other breathing-related conditions that are not necessarily caused by stoppages of breathing (apneas) but can be associated with them.

HYPOXEMIA

Hypoxemia refers to low oxygen in the blood and can be caused by a lack of effectiveness of the lungs; either the lungs are not able to "pull in" oxygen from the air or once the oxygen does get into the lungs it is not able to be passed into the blood. While the hard-core details of hypoxemia are complex, the thing to remember is that chronic obstructive pulmonary disease (COPD), severe asthma, morbid obesity, neurologic illness, sleep apnea (both obstructive and central), and very high altitudes can result in hypoxemia.

Long term, hypoxemia can result in heart failure, an excess of red blood cells in the circulation (not a good thing in most cases), delayed growth in children, problems with neurological development, and impaired sleep quality with frequent awakenings. Severe hypoxemia can lead to respiratory failure and death. Depending on the cause, treatment may include the use of supplemental oxygen (as in COPD), CPAP, or VPAP (in the case of OSA or CSA); weight loss (sometimes involving bariatric surgery); or another type of airway pressure treatment called bi-level positive airway pressure (BPAP), discussed in the following section.

HYPOVENTILATION

Hypoventilation (sometimes referred to respiratory depression) occurs when the lungs are unable to get rid of the carbon dioxide in the blood. Carbon dioxide is a waste product of our body's metabolism, and needs to be eliminated with each breath. As in the case of hypoxemia, the causes of hypoventilation are varied and include things such as neurologic illness (like Lou Gehrig's disease), certain medications or illicit drugs (like opiates or benzodiazepine medications when taken in excess), or morbid obesity (a condition known as obesity-hypoventilation syndrome).

Long term, hypoventilation can result in raising blood pressure, cardiac arrhythmias, disorientation, lethargy, convulsions, unconsciousness, and eventually death.

The bottom line is that a lack of oxygen in the tissues and/or an increase in carbon dioxide in the blood can have bad consequences, and it is important to address them if found. One way to treat these problems is a device mentioned earlier called BPAP (the trademarked name, BiPAP, is often used interchangeably, but other companies also make BPAP devices). Like a CPAP, a BPAP delivers positive airway pressure, but it differs in that it does so on two "levels"—one for inspiration and one for exhalation. In addition to keeping the upper airway open, a BPAP helps increase the efficiency of the lungs.

UPPER-AIRWAY RESISTANCE SYNDROME

While OSA comes from actual stoppages of breathing, there is another, lesser form of a "tight" airway condition known as upper-airway resistance syndrome (UARS). In this case, the airway is not completely blocked off the way it is in OSA; rather, there is simply a smaller airway, similar to snoring. This condition is more than snoring, however, with symptoms ranging from fatigue to unrefreshing sleep to chronic pain to irritable bowel syndrome.[2] While the official diagnosis of UARS is not recognized in many sleep clinics, the symptoms may improve with CPAP, MAD, or surgery—the same treatments we use to improve OSA.

CATATHRENIA

Catathrenia is a benign condition that consists of breath holding and expiratory groans that occur during REM sleep. The sound is produced during exhalation, and therefore is different than the snoring or gasping we hear with OSA, which occurs during inhalation.

It is usually not noticed by the person producing the sound, but those who hear it may be concerned. They may hear a person take a deep breath, then hold it, followed by slow exhalation that is accompanied by a high-pitched squeak or groan. Because catathrenia is benign, we usually don't recommend anything specific to treat it, although for very disruptive cases, CPAP could potentially be used.

SUMMARY AND ACTION PLAN

CSA is a disorder consisting of repetitive stoppages of breathing, not due to a blockage of the airway (as in the case of OSA) but due to a failure of the breathing signal coming from the central nervous system. It is often seen in cases of congestive heart failure or excessive use of opiate medications, or for reasons we do not quite understand yet.

CSA is important to diagnose and treat. Aside from noting how you feel in the morning, the following should be taken into consideration if there is a possibility of CSA or any of the other conditions we discussed earlier:

- Ask your bed partner to note if it sounds like you are not trying to breathe while you are sleeping.

- If you have heart problems such as congestive heart failure, it is important to follow your doctor's orders about medications and other treatment, and to do your best to improve your overall health.
- For these and any other difficulties with breathing, the first step is a visit with a physician, who more than likely will recommend a formal evaluation in a sleep lab.
- An overnight sleep test can determine if you are suffering with OSA, CSA, or some other sleep breathing condition.
- Multiple treatments for CSA may be used, depending on the situation:

  - Taking care of the underlying condition (especially heart problems).
  - VPAP (ASV) is effective, but there is unfortunately controversy using this technology in those with heart failure.
  - Supplemental oxygen.
  - Removal of the offending substance/medication.

Because many of the conditions we went over in this chapter are not well known and not frequently discussed, it would be helpful to summarize:

- Hypoxemia refers to low oxygen in the blood and can be caused by a lack of effectiveness of the lungs, usually caused by COPD, severe asthma, morbid obesity, neurologic illness, sleep apnea (both obstructive and central), and very high altitudes. Treatment includes supplemental oxygen, some type of PAP therapy, or weight loss.
- Hypoventilation occurs when the lungs are unable to get rid of the carbon dioxide in the blood, the result of neurologic illness, certain medications, illicit drugs, or morbid obesity. Treatment includes PAP therapy or weight loss.
- UARS refers to a condition where the airway is small, but not small enough for OSA to be present. Symptoms can be managed with treatments similar to OSA.
- Catathrenia is a benign condition that consists of breath holding and expiratory groans. We usually don't do anything specific to

treat it. For very disruptive cases, CPAP could potentially be used.

8

MOVIN' IN THE NIGHT, PART I

The Legs

Sleep-related movement disorders include restless legs syndrome (RLS) and periodic limb movements of sleep (PLMS), among other disorders that we will discuss in chapter 9. They are very real conditions and can be quite disturbing to sleep. Through the chapter, I will refer to each condition separately, or as a combination ("RLS/PLMS"), because they often occur together and are treated in a similar way.

RLS is also known as Willis-Ekbom disease, after the men who first described it in the medical literature. I know it sounds like a joke or a silly condition, but talk to anyone who has it—or the bed partner of someone who does—and you'll be told it is anything but funny.

Patients who have RLS report they feel an unrelenting need to move their legs, kick their legs, or get up and walk around. This obviously prevents them from being able to fall asleep or stay asleep. It can go on for hours, and it can be hell. Strange as it may sound, RLS is relatively common, affecting as much as 5–15 percent of the population, but there is often a several-year gap from the time symptoms first start to actual diagnosis.[1]

RLS symptoms can be described as anywhere from mild to incredibly severe, to the point of causing many nights of sleep deprivation, and the symptoms may gradually worsen over time.

We don't have an actual test for RLS. It's more of a clinical diagnosis, which means that the doctor bases the diagnosis on various patient-reported symptoms. For RLS, there are four main criteria, known by the acronym "URGE":

- The "U" is for "Urge." Patients say they have the urge to move their legs, usually affecting the lower half of the legs. Sometimes they'll describe it as a "creepy, crawly" feeling, an itchy feeling, or they say it feels like their legs are being pulled.
- Symptoms typically come on strong when people are at rest, the "R" of the acronym. If they're moving around throughout the day, or if they're walking around or getting up and going from place to place, they usually have no problems. It's when they lie down that it becomes troublesome.
- The "G" is for go, because if the person suffering with RLS gets up and starts moving around, the symptoms get better.
- The "E" refers to the fact that evening is predominantly when the symptoms occur. Typically, patients with RLS will be symptom free during the day, particularly if they are moving around and active. Once evening arrives, the symptoms come back.

Why is RLS so bad? Because it can prevent someone from falling asleep or from sleeping well. Additionally, in many cases, patients with RLS will be kicking throughout the night. We call these PLMS, or periodic limb movements of sleep, and they can cause difficulty staying asleep. Also, what's not usually mentioned is that patients with RLS have high rates of depression and anxiety disorders.[2]

Where does RLS come from? In most cases, the cause is unknown, but there seems to be a genetic component.[3] Additionally, certain conditions can bring it on, such as pregnancy,[4] particularly in the last trimester. Alcohol may worsen the symptoms. Sleep deprivation also may aggravate or trigger RLS symptoms. Disruptors of sleep such as OSA can make it very difficult to treat RLS if the OSA itself is not treated. If I see a patient with OSA and RLS, I will most likely start by treating the OSA first, and that alone may help at least a little with the RLS.

With that as background, let's step back for a moment and take a look at John's story.

> I'm seventy-four. About three and a half years ago, I started to have sleep problems. Specifically, restless legs, which manifested itself in spasms in my legs that would move throughout my entire body. The

RLS got worse and worse during the night and then started happening during the day.

My father had the exact same thing, maybe even worse. He would kick my mother, not realizing it because he stayed asleep. Mom would wake up black and blue, and eventually they had to get separate beds. Obviously, there is an inherited quality to RLS.

There was one thing that helped at first: chocolate. Oddly enough, somehow or other my body knew what it needed to deal with the spasms. I don't know if it was the chocolate itself, the sugar, or what. I can't explain it. I just felt the need for chocolate, and it helped.

Somewhere around this point I went to see Dr. Barone. I spent a night at the Weill Cornell Sleep Center, and the results of the sleep study were depressing. I thought I was just waking up five or six times a night, but the tests showed that I was having as many as 120 spasms an hour.

Dr. Barone initially prescribed ropinirole (Requip), which had been effective for my father. It worked for me for a little while, and then stopped working. Dr. Barone then prescribed pramipexole (Mirapex), which is something used to treat Parkinson's. It worked for a while and then it too stopped working.

Most articles I read said that people with RLS need higher levels of iron and magnesium. I went that route, but it didn't help. I went to another sleep specialist, who did a second overnight sleep study. He concluded that I had slight apnea and suggested that I should get a CPAP machine. I did and found it to be terribly awkward and I eventually sent it back.

I tried all sorts of medications, including benzodiazepines, gabapentin (Neurontin), and zolpidem (Ambien), and they didn't help. The only way I could get back to sleep after a spasm was by smoking marijuana, but I hated it.

Then I read an article in the *RLS.org Bulletin* about methadone, which is an opioid-analog used to treat pain and a detoxification agent used to help people get off cocaine and heroin. I went back to Dr. Barone at that point. We discussed it, and he prescribed a small, 5 mg dose of methadone. I needed 10 mg for a while, but then I went back to 5 mg because I wanted to take as little as possible.

I'm now taking 2.5 mg of methadone every night. I take chocolate every once in awhile. I still wake up in the middle of the night with what some people call the heebie-jeebies. I'll take another methadone 2.5 mg pill at that point, and that lets me get back to sleep. I can't tell you what a thrill it is to get a full night's sleep. I feel like a new person, getting a full night's sleep after years of having nothing but interrupted sleep, which studies show is worse than no sleep at all.

I'm getting a good night's sleep these days, seven to eight hours. I get up feeling good. I exercise in the morning and I go about doing my thing. I almost hate to say it, but I think I've got it licked.

John's story touches on some typical and some not-so-typical issues surrounding RLS. He points out that RLS can get worse with time, and the fact that his father had it strongly suggests that it may have a genetic component. Other important things to consider:

- Chocolate is not something that is generally talked about for treating RLS. However, one of the well-known treatments for RLS is engaging in an activity that takes the person's mind off the symptoms—things like doing crossword puzzles or playing video games. It is possible that John's enjoyment of chocolate may be keeping his mind occupied.
- As is true with people who have OSA, those who have PLMS (which happen in sleep) may not be aware of how often it is happening. As in the case of OSA, an in-lab test is the only definitive way to find out.
- The two medications John mentions, ropinirole (Requip) and pramipexole (Mirapex), are both used in treating Parkinson's disease. It is important to point out that RLS and PLMS do *not* have a major relationship to Parkinson's disease (although patients with Parkinson's disease can also suffer from RLS and PLMS). People who look up these medications online may become unnecessarily concerned (if they just have RLS/PLMS).
- John mentions his iron levels. Doctors can check a measure of iron stores in the blood called ferritin. The normal level ranges approximately between 15 and 300, but less than 50 is considered low in someone who has RLS/PLMS. Young women may often have low ferritin simply because of their monthly menstruation. But regardless of the reason, a reading at this level in people with RLS/PLMS may actually *be* the reason for their RLS/PLMS. Replacing iron with certain foods and taking iron supplements may improve the symptoms over time (months).

- Examples of iron-rich foods include red meat; egg yolks; dark, leafy greens (like spinach or collards); dried fruit (like prunes or raisins); liver; and artichokes.
- As for the iron pills, there are many brands and types. We usually have patients start with one pill per day for a week or so, increasing one pill per day for another week, ending with three pills per day by the third week, continuing on for a few months. After several months, we will recheck the ferritin level to see if it has gone up, and ideally the patient will be able to tell if the symptoms have improved. Taking iron pills like this can lead to constipation, so I always ask my patients to take them with prune juice. The prune juice will offset the constipation, and the vitamin C in the juice actually helps to absorb iron.
- Vitamin B12, if low, may also contribute to RLS/PLMS, and replacing it may improve symptoms.
- Magnesium is less well studied, but taking magnesium pills may relax the central nervous system and possibly reduce RLS/PLMS.
- A new and safe way of treating RLS is with what is known as "counter-stimulation." The principle here is that some sort of vibration or pressure is applied to the legs, which reduces the symptoms of RLS. The Relaxis pad—a vibrating pad that is placed under the sheets near the legs—is one such device.
- Other alternative treatments for RLS exist, including medical marijuana, which is a hot topic in the neurology world. Someday, it may be used as a treatment for RLS. For now, it is not. As I have said before, I like treatment options that are (1) safe and (2) may work.
- Methadone has a big stigma, given its association as a treatment for heroin addiction. However, there is data showing a low dose of methadone can be helpful in RLS.[5] It is an opiate pain medication, and the thought is that methadone reduces the feelings of discomfort known to occur in RLS. In John's case, I figured it was worth a try given our failure with the other, more conservative approaches.
- Because of methadone's power, I am restricting John from using any other prescription medication along with it, and it has been working well for him. One concern all doctors have with methadone (and all opiates in general) is the potential for addiction.

However, when given in small doses and taken only as prescribed, the risk for addiction is extremely low.

As John's history suggests, RLS is treated in a variety of ways. I like to start with a conservative treatment, which consists of avoiding caffeine, nicotine, alcohol, and certain medications (especially antihistamines like diphenhydramine [Benadryl]). I had a patient who was taking Benadryl for itching and for what she thought was insomnia. It turned out that the Benadryl was actually aggravating her RLS. We stopped the Benadryl and her RLS improved.

Stretching before bed can be very helpful for dealing with RLS. I recommend a leg stretch for my patients in which I have them stand up against a wall at an angle, so their calves are stretched. I have them do five sets of holding this stretch for thirty seconds, interspersed with a few seconds of rest between each set.

Taking hot or cold baths, whirlpool baths, applying hot or cold packs, limb massage, or vibratory or electrical stimulation of the feet and toes before bedtime may be of use. Relaxation techniques can also help.

Importantly, any underlying medical conditions—such as diabetes, nutritional deficiencies, kidney disease, thyroid disease, varicose veins, arthritis, back or knee problems, nerve damages (called neuropathy) or Parkinson's disease—can bring on or worsen RLS.

Let's talk about RLS in pregnancy again. During pregnancy there is a two- to three-times higher chance that women will experience RLS. The likelihood of having RLS increases over the course of the pregnancy, as does the severity of symptoms, with the highest being at the seventh to eighth month.[6] The good news is that 70 percent of those with RLS will enjoy significant improvement or complete remission shortly after delivery.

The reasons for RLS in pregnancy are not fully understood. Problems with iron and folate, genetic susceptibility, high estrogen levels, and the stretching or compression of nerves have been proposed, but the evidence is not clear.[7] While medications listed below can be used to treat very severe cases, most doctors prefer to treat the symptoms conservatively given the potential for risk to the fetus. This includes iron supplements (if low), exercise, and stretching. Simply knowing that the symptoms should improve once the child is born can also be a relieving factor.[8]

The use of daily medication is usually reserved for patients who have RLS/PLMS frequently rather than for situations in which the symptoms are simply bothersome every now and then. In these cases, we can use them on an as-needed basis. The medications used in RLS may help with the symptoms, but they do not cure it. Over time, some medications may become less effective, or we may need to shift them around. Here is a list of ones we typically use:

- *Dopamine-based.* These are medications that are primarily used to treat Parkinson's disease, even though, as I said, RLS/PLMS does not lead to Parkinson's disease. The medications come in pill form—ropinirole (Requip), pramipexole (Mirapex), carbidopa/levodopa (Sinemet)—and in a patch, rotigotine (Neupro). They are usually tolerated well but can have side effects including nausea and dizziness. These types of medications are considered among the first line, but I personally tend to reserve them for later use if we need them.
- The problem with dopamine-related products is what may happen long term. They can cause what is known as augmentation, which is a progressive worsening of the RLS symptoms, including symptom onset earlier in the day until finally they occur around-the-clock and/or move into the arms or even the torso. Removing the person from all dopamine-related products can solve the problem, although that can be uncomfortable in and of itself as the RLS/PLMS symptoms return. Typically we add another medication as we are weaning or cutting a patient off dopamine-based medications.
- Another important thing to understand is that dopamine medications can lead to compulsive behaviors like shopping or gambling; stopping the medication can reverse the behavior.
- *Gabapentin-based.* GABA is a molecule produced in the central nervous system that "slows things down." A medication known as gabapentin (Neurontin) promotes this slowing down of the central nervous system. While technically an antiseizure medication, gabapentin is used by neurologists and other doctors for a variety of issues, including pain, headaches, and RLS.
- Gabapentin is my personal first-line treatment because the side effects are usually not severe and the long-term problems that

plague the dopamine-based medications are not an issue. Side effects may include dizziness, fatigue, and sleepiness, the last of which can be helpful in cases of sleep disturbance or insomnia. Two relatives of gabapentin—gabapentin enacarbil (Hortizant) and pregabalin (Lyrica)—may also be useful or, in some cases, even more effective than gabapentin.

- *Benzodiazepines.* These are medications for insomnia, which we discussed in chapter 4. They also work on the GABA system and can treat many different conditions, including anxiety and muscle spasm. They can be very helpful when used in the right patient. The problem with these medications is that they often cause daytime sleepiness and potential addiction, although this is low when used as prescribed. The other potential issue, which we discussed earlier, is that they can worsen OSA.

- Depending on the situation, I also may prescribe opiates (as I did with John), but this is usually reserved for special or difficult cases.

PERIODIC LIMB MOVEMENTS OF SLEEP/PERIODIC LIMB MOVEMENT DISORDER

PLMS typically occur in someone who has RLS, which is why I listed them together as RLS/PLMS throughout this chapter. Unlike RLS, we actually do have a test for PLMS, which is an overnight sleep test. Symptoms range from a small amount of movement in the ankles and toes to the frank kicking of legs (less commonly, the arms can move). A bed partner may report these, but many times the patient is not aware of suffering from them. If the limb movements cause sleep disruption or result in unrefreshing sleep, we refer to the condition as periodic limb movement disorder (PLMD).

More than 80 percent of people with RLS also experience PLMS.[9] The movements occur in spurts every five to ninety seconds, and can be disruptive to the patient as well as the bed partner. Someone with PLMD often also suffers daytime sleepiness. PLMD is estimated to occur in approximately 4 percent of adults, but is more common in older folks, especially women.[10]

Like RLS, we are not sure what causes PLMS/PLMD. It is seen in patients with conditions such as narcolepsy, OSA, and heart disease, and in those involved in shift work. The use of caffeine, alcohol, or nicotine can make them worse. Same goes for stress. The way to treat PLMS or PLMD is similar to the way we treat RLS. John's case was actually PLMD, as he did not report RLS symptoms. But, as you can see, we treat both essentially the same way.

Something I would like to point out here is that bed partners may say that they see "leg twitching" during the night. This can be completely benign. It also could be seizures (discussed below) or signs of PLMS. A sleep test will help us figure it out.

NOCTURNAL LEG CRAMPS

I also want to briefly mention nocturnal leg cramps, which often occur because of dehydration or some sort of electrolyte imbalance. Hydrating throughout the day is important for many reasons (drink your eight glasses) and can aid in the prevention of cramps. Water is the liquid of choice but something like Gatorade or tonic water can work. If the cramps persist, a visit to a doctor would be helpful.

SUMMARY AND ACTION PLAN

There are many ways to deal with RLS/PLMS, including medications and natural approaches. To summarize:

- If you have RLS, usually you will experience the four "URGE" criteria. Talk to your doctor.
- Treating any underlying condition like nerve problems can be helpful.
- Altering or removing some medications or substances (like Benadryl) can also provide a benefit.
- Have your iron levels checked, especially ferritin. If low, you should try an iron supplement (if okayed by your doctor). Same with vitamin B12.
- Try the calf stretch before bed.

- Doing distracting activities before bed such as crossword puzzles can keep your mind off the symptoms and make it easier to fall asleep. Video games or a conversation with your spouse at bedtime can be effective.
- Medications include the dopamine drugs and the non-dopamine drugs, as well as others. A conversation with your doctor would help to decide which ones to try in light of how severe and how often your symptoms occur.
- Find out from your bed partner if you are kicking your legs throughout the night, and if it seems to wake you up. This may be a sign of periodic limb movements of sleep (PLMS), which often goes along with RLS. A sleep test is needed for confirmation.
- Nocturnal leg cramps usually happen in the setting of dehydration or electrolyte imbalance. Make sure you are drinking enough water throughout the day. If the cramps happen frequently and do not get better, a visit to a doctor and a blood check may be needed.

9

MOVIN' IN THE NIGHT, PART II

The Parasomnias

Parasomnias is a term that covers all forms of abnormal movements and sensations that occur near to or during sleep. It includes all forms of sleepwalking, REM behavior disorder (RBD), and even stranger things like sexsomnia and exploding head syndrome. Some of the parasomnias, like *hypnagogic* and *hypnopompic* hallucinations, we cover in chapters 3 and 10 and will not be talked about here. Other abnormal movements in sleep, like seizures, will be covered here, even though, by strict definition, they are not parasomnias. In any case, please read on. This is a fascinating topic.

The best way to examine parasomnias is to break them down into ones that occur during REM sleep and ones occurring in non-REM (NREM) sleep. Let's start with the REM parasomnias. They include RBD, sleep paralysis, and nightmares.

REM BEHAVIOR DISORDER

During REM sleep, there is normally a paralysis of our muscles, which is to prevent us from acting out our dreams (see the discussion in chapter 2). In RBD, the prevailing thought is that an area of the brain stem (in the upper neck region) is not working properly.

When all is going well, messages telling us to move are created in our brain and then travel down the spinal cord into the nerves that control the muscles of the body. In normal REM sleep, the signals from the brain to move the muscles are stopped, which basically puts us into a state of paralysis so we do not act out our dreams. In RBD, however, there is *behavior* in REM sleep, when there shouldn't be; the signals coming from the brain move down to the muscles and activate them. This can lead to striking a bed partner, punching the walls, or in some cases falling out of bed.

RBD is typically a condition of older men, and the classic scenario is an elderly gentleman showing up at the sleep clinic with a wife who has a black eye. This is because he had a dream where he was boxing and ended up hitting his wife in the dream. RBD is dangerous in that there is potential for someone to hurt themselves or the bed partner, but the real reason we care about it is because it can be associated with a form of chronic disease called synucleinopathies.

Synucleinopathies are diseases in which abnormal proteins build up in the brain. They include Parkinson's disease, dementia with Lewy bodies, and multiple-system atrophy. They are known as neurodegenerative diseases, and unfortunately there is no way of stopping them once they start. According to the medical literature, 40 to 75 percent of people diagnosed with RBD will develop one of these conditions within ten years.[1] This is a difficult topic to discuss with patients, but I tell them—as I tell you now—that I am not sure I believe the numbers.

By that I mean the person who makes it to a doctor is one who strikes his bed partner or falls out of bed in the context of having acted out during a violent dream. But let's say there is a woman whose dream is simply picking flowers in the garden. Her acting out may not lead to any noticeable behavior during sleep. This has not been proven, but I suspect that more people than we think may have RBD, which in turn makes the possibility of developing a synucleinopathy lower than what is reported. Again, these are my own thoughts, and not necessarily fact.

Regardless, all we can do now is treat the symptoms of RBD. Treatments include high doses of melatonin (3 to 12 mg), low doses (0.25 to 0.5 mg) of clonazepam (Klonopin), or a combination of the two. Both have been shown to work in reducing the actual acting out of dreams, but no one is really sure why they work.

We mentioned that RBD tends to happen in older men, and that there is a risk for some unfortunate consequences. But other situations in which RBD may be seen include psychiatric disease (like posttraumatic stress disorder), use of antidepressant medications (the SSRIs like sertraline [Zoloft] or paroxetine [Paxil]), already having Parkinson's disease, or having narcolepsy. Finally, there are some cases of obstructive sleep apnea (OSA) where the patients seem to be acting out their dreams when in fact they are experiencing the effect of the brain and body partially waking up from the stoppages of breathing; the term for this is called *pseudo-RBD*—"pseudo" because the OSA is causing the symptoms.

Fortunately, RBD is an area of active research, one in which I am personally involved. In time, I am confident that the physicians and scientists in our field will uncover more information as to why RBD happens and what we can do about it.

I am also hopeful that we will soon see the development of reliable neuroprotective agents, which are substances or medications that can be taken to prevent or lessen the likelihood of nervous system injury from occurring. Ideally, if we find RBD in someone, we would be able to give them a neuroprotective agent and possibly prevent something like Parkinson's disease from happening in the future. But this, of course, remains to be seen.

SLEEP PARALYSIS

Sleep paralysis is a condition that occurs when a person awakes from REM sleep. As I mentioned earlier, in REM sleep our muscles are completely paralyzed. Sleep paralysis may occur because the person is basically awake but the body is still "in" REM sleep, and thus paralyzed. There may be dream imagery that feels real (again, from REM sleep) in the partially awakened person, and the person's feeling of paralysis may be frightening.

This has actually been thought to be an explanation for why people report they have been abducted by aliens. Sleep paralysis can happen to anybody, and although it is scary, it is usually totally benign. But if it happens frequently (once per week, for example), it could be a sign of

OSA or narcolepsy, and it probably should be evaluated further if other symptoms of these conditions are noted.

NIGHTMARES

Nightmares are vivid dreams with intense feelings of fear or dread, sometimes in the setting of seeing or hearing something frightening or anxiety provoking, that cause us to awaken out of REM sleep as a result. Because periods of REM sleep become progressively longer as the night progresses, a nightmare will most often occur in the early morning hours.

Reassurance is all that is usually needed, but reducing stress levels, keeping bedtime routines that are relaxing, and ensuring adequate rest are all potential treatments. If nightmares happen repeatedly, a referral to a sleep specialist may be needed. Medications or other psychological treatments may be required, especially in cases where posttraumatic stress may be involved.

The NREM parasomnias include sleepwalking, night terrors, confusional arousals, sleep eating, sleep sex, exploding head syndrome, teeth grinding, and others. They may be triggered in certain individuals by alcohol, sleep deprivation, physical activity, emotional stress, depression, medications, fever, or other sleep conditions. I will also briefly mention nighttime seizures.

SLEEPWALKING

One of my favorite movies of all time is the 2008 comedy *Step Brothers*. In it, the characters portrayed by John C. Reilly and Will Ferrell are forty-somethings who, among other problems, suffer from sleepwalking. It is very funny to see it in the movie and, believe or not, there is some truth to how it is portrayed.

Sleepwalking is quite common in childhood, especially around the ages of eleven to twelve, but it is experienced by only about 4 percent of adults (the two men in *Step Brothers* were among this unfortunate 4 percent). It usually happens when people are transitioning from N2 sleep into N3 sleep. (To reiterate, N2 is the baseline of our sleep, while

N3 is very deep sleep.) The reason children experience sleepwalking more often than adults is because they tend to spend more time in N3.

Sleepwalking, however, can also be associated with certain specific conditions. Anything that disrupts sleep can potentially lead to sleepwalking. If someone spends a lot of time in N3 (those who are chronically sleep deprived, for example), there is a higher likelihood of sleepwalking.

In some cases, people who have been prescribed zolpidem (Ambien) or eszopiclone (Lunesta), among other sleep aids, report sleepwalking.[2] What happens is that these medications obviously put a person to sleep. Once asleep, if the person is awakened by something internally (like OSA) or externally (like a noise), he or she may only be partially awake. In this partially awakened state, people may get up in the middle of the night, jump into the car, and go out for a drive. Or more sinister things like attacking their bed partner may occur.

What's fascinating about sleepwalking is that certain areas of the brain are shut off while others are actually still working. The frontal lobes are the areas of the brain that provide a "filter" that prevents us from "bad behaviors." When people sleepwalk, the frontal lobes are still asleep but other areas of the brain that know how to walk around the house, open a door, or even operate a car are awake. This allows people to move about in their environment without actually knowing what they're doing. People say that one should never wake a sleepwalker up in the middle of their walking. The reason for this is that since the frontal lobes are asleep, any kind of sudden movement (such as would occur when abruptly awakening a person) may be perceived as a threat. And because the frontal lobes are asleep, the filter to not attack someone who's trying to help has been turned off. As a result, the sleepwalker could do harm to himself or herself or someone else. For example, reports have described sleepwalkers leaving the house, driving a car, and even firing a loaded gun.[3]

What to do about sleepwalking? If there is a possibility of another sleep condition, it should be addressed first. Like RBD, the key thing to focus on is bedtime safety, including locked doors/windows, taking knobs off ovens and stoves, and so on. And reassurance. But as I said earlier, finding out if there's another sleep issue (like OSA) and treating it will usually help with the problem. Sometimes medications may be needed—or, in the case of some of the sleep aids we mentioned, they may need to be eliminated or changed to something else. Otherwise, simply guiding the sleepwalker back to bed with reassuring statements can be helpful.

SLEEP-RELATED EATING DISORDER

Sleep-related eating disorder—sleep eating or somnambulistic eating—is a form of sleepwalking. In these cases, patients often report unexplained weight gain or evidence of eating in sleep (crumbs in the bed, food wrappers from food not remembered being eaten, and the like). The way to deal with sleep eating is similar to how we deal with other forms of sleepwalking. It begins with treating any underlying sleep conditions, like OSA or restless legs syndrome,[4] and discontinuing the use of offending agents, like zolpidem (Ambien).[5] If more is needed, dopaminergic drugs (like those used in restless legs syndrome) or the antiseizure medication topiramate (Topamax) is sometimes used.[6]

SEXSOMNIA

Sexsomnia is what it sounds like—a condition in which people engage in sexual activity while being asleep. It is essentially a form of sleepwalking, and the same information we talked about regarding sleepwalking applies to sexsomnia. As one can imagine, this condition has tremendous potential forensic implications—cases of sexual assault and rape, for example.[7]

EXPLODING HEAD SYNDROME

First reported in the 1890s, this is a benign condition described as hearing loud imagined sounds (like an exploding bomb) when falling asleep or waking up.[8] The cause is not known, but theories include the brain not shutting down completely, disrupted sleep, stress and anxiety, or parts of the inner workings of the ear shifting suddenly. Certain types of medications can be used to treat the problem, but typically reassurance is enough.

CONFUSIONAL AROUSALS

In the sleep world, an arousal is like a partial awakening. Confusional arousals are another benign condition during which an individual has a partial awakening from sleep and remains in a confused state. The people usually remain in bed as they sit up and look around, and then return to sleep. The arousals last anywhere from seconds to minutes. As with most conditions of this nature, the thing to look out for during a confusional arousal is another sleep disorder that may be triggering it. Like sleepwalking, they are relatively common in kids, and become less so in adults.

SLEEP TERRORS (NIGHT TERRORS)

Sleep terrors are among the most disruptive sleep disorders, since they usually result in loud screams and what *seems* like extreme panic. They typically occur in children, and what is really interesting is that the child is actually not having a nightmare and has no recollection of the event. Because of this fact, observers (in this case the parents) tend to be shaken up, whereas the actual screamer does not recall being scared. This differentiates sleep terrors from nightmares: Following a nightmare, the child will give a very detailed account of the dream and seek to be consoled by the parent. In sleep terrors, the child is very difficult to wake up (because the child is in deep sleep, that N3 sleep we spoke of before) and cannot be consoled.

As with sleepwalking, children tend to outgrow sleep terrors. If they occur commonly, one effective technique would be to wake the child up preemptively, typically fifteen to thirty minutes before the sleep terror usually takes place. In cases in which the symptoms are severe (especially when present in adults), an overnight sleep test or further sleep evaluation may be warranted. Medications or other treatments may also be required.

TEETH GRINDING/CLENCHING (BRUXISM)

According to the bible of the sleep world, *The International Classification of Sleep Disorders—Third Edition* (ICSD-3), bruxism is not technically categorized as a parasomnia, but I put it here because it makes sense. This is a common sleep disorder in which people grind or clench their teeth through the night. It can result in waking with headaches, temporomandibular joint pain, or dental issues. While it can be seen by itself, it usually presents in cases with anxiety or compulsive issues. Also, people with OSA may have bruxism; they may be moving their jaw in an attempt to open their airway, which results in the teeth mashing against each other. The way to treat bruxism is with a mouth guard to protect the teeth and/or to identify and deal with the underlying condition—treatment of anxiety, for example, or identification and treatment of OSA.

NOCTURNAL SEIZURES

Like bruxism, nocturnal seizures are not considered parasomnias, but they fit in well with this category, which is why I have included them here. Nocturnal seizures can be frightening to witness—the shaking and writhing that is characteristic of a classic seizure—but they may also be more subtle, such as moving the arms or turning the head to one side or another while staying in one position.

These signs tend to help us differentiate nocturnal seizures from conditions like confusional arousals, which tend to be varied in terms of the actual action that is taking place. With nocturnal seizures, the movements tend to be what are called *stereotyped*, in that sufferers may make the same repetitive motions over and over and over again (like moving the arm or hand).

Additionally, people with nocturnal seizures may wake up feeling very tired. The way to treat nocturnal seizures is with antiseizure medications and making sure that other sleep issues are addressed. If there is any possibility of nocturnal seizures or, as is often the case, there is a possibility of other abnormal movements (such as REM behavior disorder or sleepwalking), an overnight sleep test would be of use and potentially aid the doctor to discover what is actually occurring.

As a corollary to this, some patients tell me their bed partner says that they are twitching throughout the night. Involuntary twitching may be a manifestation of seizures when awake, but it may represent many different things when someone is sleeping. It could be the PLMS we talked about in the preceding chapter or one of the other parasomnias described above.

To end this chapter, I'd like to review some of the "normal" conditions we all experience from time to time—specifically, sleep talking and sleep starts.

SLEEP TALKING

It has been reported that as many as two-thirds of us have talked in our sleep. It really is a benign condition, but like the rest of the conditions we spoke about in this chapter, if it happens frequently, if it disrupts a person's sleep or their bed partner's sleep, or if there is the possibility of another problem (like OSA), it would be useful to see a sleep specialist.

SLEEP STARTS

We have all experienced sleep starts. They go by many names, such as hypnic jerk, hypnagogic jerk, sleep twitch, or night start. They are basically involuntary twitches that occur just as a person is beginning to fall asleep, kind of like a hiccup. They can cause the person to awaken suddenly for a brief time, which may interrupt sleep in some cases. Sleep starts may also be accompanied by a falling sensation. While sleep starting is typically a benign condition, it may be a sign of poor sleep quality or quantity.

SUMMARY AND ACTION PLAN

The term *parasomnia* encompasses all forms of abnormal movements and sensations that occur near to or during sleep, and they are broken down into those occurring in REM sleep and those occurring in NREM sleep. We also went over conditions, such as nocturnal seizures, that are not necessarily parasomnias by definition but can impact sleep and overall health.

- With all of these, the most important consideration is *safety*. This includes making sure the bed and bed environment are safe (doors and windows locked, bed area padded with couch cushions to break a fall, etc.).
- Many of the issues can be related to another sleep problem. If you experience any of these abnormal activities in the night and feel that your sleep is disrupted, or if you feel tired and hungover in the morning or are disturbing your bed partner, it would be a good idea to see a sleep specialist.

Here are some additional thoughts on the subject:

- With many of these problems, a regular sleep-wake schedule can be helpful, as can getting enough sleep at night.
- Tell your doctor about all medications and substances you are taking. Some of these (like zolpidem [Ambien]) can be a trigger.
- Stress reduction and avoidance of alcohol, nicotine, and similar substances are important.
- Keeping a journal of when these abnormal movements occur can help you and your doctor devise a plan to discover what may be triggering them.
- Bedroom safety is most important in preventing accidents.
- A sleep test can help with the diagnosis.
- Depending on what is found, either treating the underlying condition (such as OSA) or medication can be the way to go.

10

NARCOLEPSY
Being Too Sleepy

The way narcolepsy is portrayed in movies and TV shows is entertaining but hardly accurate. The character on the screen is usually in the middle of an activity of one sort or another, and all of a sudden he or she falls asleep with no warning whatsoever. Yes, there is a possibility of this happening, but in real life it's not usually the case.

Narcolepsy is a disorder characterized by excessive sleepiness and several other symptoms. Typically, people with narcolepsy will start having these symptoms in their early to middle teen years. They may find themselves falling asleep in class or while doing homework, prompting the people around them to react by saying they are lazy.

The term *narcolepsy* was coined in 1880 by the French physician Jean-Baptiste-Édouard Gélineau, who combined the Greek words *narkē*, which means "sleep" or "numbness," with *lepsis*, which means "attack."[1] However, perhaps the first time that narcolepsy was described in any setting was in Dante Alighieri's *Divine Comedy*, composed between 1307 and his death in 1321. In it, Dante complains that he is very sleepy, and he reports experiencing short and refreshing naps, visions and hallucinations, and episodes of muscle weakness and falls, which are always triggered by strong emotions. We will be seeing throughout this chapter that these symptoms form the main criteria for the diagnosis of narcolepsy.[2]

While less than 1 percent of the population actually has narcolepsy, it is common enough, and most people know someone who has it. It is also very treatable. Importantly, there is usually a ten-year gap from the time people start having symptoms to the time they are diagnosed. That was true for one of my patients, Linda, who first had symptoms of narcolepsy when she was seven or eight.

Looking back on it now, there were signs I had problems with sleep all my life, but it was a long time before I was able to put the pieces together. Things started to get rough when I was in high school. I would fall asleep in class in the morning and I would drag myself around the rest of the day. I figured I just wasn't getting enough sleep and everyone, including the doctors I saw, would say, yeah, you're a growing teenager, and that's the way it is.

It wasn't until my junior year in college that I saw it for what it really was. I was taking a speech class. My partner in the class had narcolepsy, and that was the subject of the speech she was working on. As we practiced our speeches, I sat there listening to her, dumbfounded, and said, "Oh, my God, that's me. That's exactly how I feel. Every day. The same symptoms."

I ended up seeing a sleep specialist, going through an extensive sleep study and that was it. They diagnosed me and said I had narcolepsy.

I'm twenty-four years old now. The earliest I can remember having symptoms was probably when I was seven or eight. But as I understand it, narcolepsy is diagnosed late in life for most people. You're tired but everyone you know is tired. I was nineteen or twenty before I actually went to a sleep doctor and had a sleep test.

When the doctor suspects narcolepsy, the sleep test is a two-parter. You begin by spending the night in a typical sleep test with wires hooked up to all parts of your body. The next day, when you wake, they have you take a series of five naps. For me, that was the easy part. If I'm not on medication, you can tell me to go to sleep and I'll fall asleep in a matter of minutes. In other words, during the second part of the test, I was able to slide right into those naps. It was actually harder to stay awake when they tried to keep me from going back to sleep.

I have seen various doctors over the years, including a psychiatrist who misdiagnosed me and put me on ADHD medication during my sophomore year of college. I had a tough time staying awake during morning classes, but nobody I saw had a good understanding of narcolepsy. It's kind of a rare thing. Dr. Barone is the only narcolepsy specialist I've seen. He looked at the sleep study and confirmed the diagnosis.

They treat it in various ways, including giving you stimulants to keep you awake. That was the first thing we tried. Medications like amphetamine salts (Adderall) or lisdexamfetamine (Vyvanse), which I'm currently on. They keep me awake and allow me to function normally.

At one point, to help me sleep better, Dr. Barone tried a medication called Xyrem. It's a crazy sort of thing—an FDA-approved form of gamma-hydroxybutyrate, which is the date rape drug. I was on it for about four months. I had good luck with it, but unfortunately the side effects were too much. It's a heavy-duty medication and I had to stop.

Right now I'm just on medications during the day. I take an over-the-counter sleeping pill when I go to bed so I don't constantly wake up during the night. For the most part, the combination seems to be working, but it's a constant struggle. It never feels like I'm 100 percent right. From time to time it gets to me, but for the most part I lead a successful, normal life.

Dr. Barone and I decided that from Monday through Friday, when I'm at work, I would take an extended-release stimulant first thing in the morning. On weekends, if I'm not doing anything terribly complicated or demanding, I can just take an instant-release medication during the day.

Am I depressed by the fact I have narcolepsy? Not really. I've had it since I was young, and it was almost a relief when I was diagnosed and suddenly there was an explanation for why I feel the way I do. I don't let it get to me now because I don't really know any other way. I don't know any time when I wasn't exhausted, so for me it's just kind of life.

At the same time, I don't want to downplay the seriousness or debilitating nature of narcolepsy. A lot of people don't understand it and are quick to brush it off as a mild inconvenience. I have a good job and I go to work every day, but narcolepsy is a really tough condition to deal with on a daily basis. I wouldn't be able to function normally without the medications, but they come with side effects that can be very taxing on the body and mind.

Linda's history provides valuable insights into many aspects of narcolepsy. We will talk more about them later in the chapter, but here are
some of my immediate thoughts.

- Sleepy people, especially teenagers, sometimes get misdiagnosed
  as having attention-deficit hyperactivity disorder (ADHD), just
  like Linda. While we can treat these problems with the same type
  of medicine (stimulants), the underlying issue in sleepy people
  (those with narcolepsy or obstructive sleep apnea, for example) is
  sleepiness, which certainly may cause difficulty with attention and
  other cognitive tasks, but is definitely not the same thing as
  ADHD.
- Stimulants are the first line of treatment in narcolepsy, but they
  come with side effects, including possibly speeding up the heart
  rate and/or raising blood pressure. Patients have also reported
  personality changes like irritability with some of these medications. But in the right patient, they can be life changing. We will
  talk more about these shortly.
- I was hoping that gamma-hydroxybutyrate (Xyrem) would be right
  for Linda, but the side effects were problematic. Nausea or vomit-
  ing, dizziness, bed-wetting, sleepwalking, or tremors are common
  side effects,[3] and it cannot be combined with alcohol or other
  sleeping pills because it can cause an unsafe reduction in breathing. Despite all this, gamma-hydroxybutyrate can be helpful, not
  only for the sleepiness of narcolepsy but it may also reduce or
  eliminate episodes of cataplexy.
- As I tell all my patients struggling with narcolepsy, the number
  one concern is safety—safety with medications, safety if they need
  to drive or operate heavy machinery, and so on. In Linda's case, if
  we can get her through the workweek, we both feel it is better to
  take it easier on the weekends in terms of medications.
- The ideal situation for someone struggling with narcolepsy would
  be to get into a routine with their sleep and medications so that
  the condition doesn't interfere with their lives. For some of my
  patients with narcolepsy, I ask them to schedule fifteen- to twenty-minute naps around lunchtime, and that short time out often
  helps them get through the day. Of course, if they work, they

would need a doctor's note for an employer, but it can make a huge difference.

- There is a genetic component to narcolepsy, but that doesn't explain all cases. As in all aspects of medicine and health, there is a *nature* component (our genes) and a *nurture* component (exposure to substances in the environment).

- I am glad Linda is not depressed, but many patients with narcolepsy can be, particularly since no one really understands the exact nature of the illness. Fortunately, there are good support groups that patients can turn to. The Narcolepsy Network—http://narcolepsynetwork.org/resources/support-groups—is a good place to start.

As I said earlier, narcolepsy consists of excessive daytime sleepiness along with other symptoms. The other symptoms include cataplexy, hallucinations, and sleep paralysis.

The *excessive daytime sleepiness* that characterizes narcolepsy cannot be attributed to medication, obstructive sleep apnea, or any other sleep disorder. In addition to falling asleep during class or during a meeting, excessive daytime sleepiness can manifest itself while driving or sitting in traffic. Patients tell me they can be at a movie or a show, and they fall asleep in the middle of the action.

The second component of narcolepsy, *cataplexy*, is a symptom in which patients lose muscle tone in their body. It often happens when someone is laughing hard or is very angry. It can present itself as something subtle, such as a cup falling out of the person's hand. In other cases the symptoms may include the head falling forward and the patient not being able to lift it up. In still others, patients' knees buckle and they lose the ability to speak clearly. In more extreme cases, patients can lose all muscle tone and may actually fall to the ground.

Patients with narcolepsy can have cataplexy, but not always. If they do have cataplexy, the episodes generally last about two minutes. In cases where someone actually falls to the ground, it is different from a seizure in that the person doesn't lose consciousness. Talking to them afterward, they may say, "I was totally awake, totally aware, I just couldn't move."

Cataplexy was first extensively studied in narcoleptic dogs. Videos of dogs with cataplexy can be found online (type "Rusty the narcoleptic dog" into a search engine for a good example), and they're fascinating: the dogs run around in an excited manner, and then just drop to the ground. They are totally fine a short while later, and the process begins again.

We think that cataplexy takes place when REM sleep intrudes onto the wakefulness state. The paralysis we see in REM sleep hits the sufferer, who all of a sudden loses muscle tone.

Patients with narcolepsy will often have *hallucinations*, which we briefly discussed in chapter 3. They may hear a sound (like a doorbell) or see something (like a slow-moving shadow) that is not actually there. This is a case of dream imagery intruding into a half-wake/half-sleep state. If the hallucinations happen when a patient is falling asleep, they are referred to as hypnogogic; when waking up, they are called hypnopompic.

In the classic case, someone will say, "I fell asleep. As I was waking up, I felt a strange presence in the room, I heard someone calling my name, and I saw a dark shadow coming at me." People who report alien abductions are probably having hypnogogic or hypnopompic hallucinations along with sleep paralysis, which is the fourth component of narcolepsy.

Patients suffering from *sleep paralysis* actually *cannot* move their bodies. This symptom can occur in the context of hallucinations, and it can be quite scary.

When a person goes into REM sleep, his or her body is completely paralyzed, head to toe, except for the eyes, the diaphragm (allowing breathing), and a very small muscle in the inner ear. Patients with narcolepsy will frequently have sleep paralysis, but the thing to remember is that everyone experiences sleep paralysis every now and then. I've had it myself. It's usually not indicative of narcolepsy as long as it's not a common occurrence.

Please note: Not all patients with narcolepsy experience all four of these symptoms. Like all facets of medicine, the textbook does not always reflect what is encountered in real life.

The hypothalamus, a particular area of the brain, controls many factors we rarely think about—factors like body temperature, hunger and sleep, and wake cycles. The hypothalamus is important in narcolepsy because it produces the hormone hypocretin (sometimes called orexin). We suspect that hypocretin is the sleep-wake stabilizer. If people are awake, it will help keep them awake; if people are asleep, it will help them stay asleep.

An important question I often get asked is: What causes narcolepsy? For the most part, we don't entirely know. Narcolepsy may have a genetic cause; many patients tell me their mother or uncle had a similar set of symptoms. It could also be caused by an autoimmune condition in which the body attacks itself following a viral illness, for example. When I suspect narcolepsy, I always ask the patient, "Was there an event you can remember that triggered these symptoms?" A viral illness is a potential cause. Head trauma is another, and there are even reports of patients developing narcolepsy after receiving the H1N1 flu vaccine.[4]

Regardless of the actual cause of narcolepsy, once these nerve cells are lost in a high enough percentage, the amount of hypocretin that is produced reaches a critically low threshold, and symptoms of narcolepsy appear.

HOW DO WE DIAGNOSE NARCOLEPSY?

A clinical history of the four components I mentioned is important. We also can do laboratory testing. Blood work can be done, looking at what's called HLA, which has to do with a person's immune system. We also have a spinal tap test that looks at hypocretin, but this is not done very commonly.

When we suspect narcolepsy, more often than not we ask the patient to come in for PSG/MSLT testing (which is a combination of the polysomnography and multiple sleep latency tests). During these tests, we're interested in learning how quickly the patient falls asleep as well as what stage of sleep he or she goes into. During the MSLT part of the test, a person who has narcolepsy will fall asleep on average in less than eight minutes in all of the five naps that the person is asked to take.

During these short naps, most patients will experience at least two periods in which they go into REM sleep. This is a sign of narcolepsy because people typically go into REM sleep only when they have been asleep for 60–120 minutes. During a 15–20 minute nap, there is no reason for REM sleep to be achieved. Interestingly, patients with narcolepsy will often say that they dream during short naps. This is because they are abnormally heading into REM sleep very quickly.

If I diagnose a patient as having narcolepsy, I'll usually start the treatment by prescribing a stimulant medication, either modafinil (Provigil) or armodafinil (Nuvigil). Modafinil has been available in the United States for twenty years or so, and its close "cousin," armodafinil, was introduced in 2007. The two medications basically help the brain and body "speed up," which, in turn, helps reduce sleepiness. I usually ask patients to take the medication during weekdays and then give themselves a break, at least for a day, on the weekend.

The main side effects of modafinil or armodafinil can be headache and stomach upset.[5] Both tend to resolve with longer use. If a woman is taking an oral contraceptive, they may reduce the pill's effectiveness. I always tell my female patients to discuss the use of contraceptives with their ob/gyn once I put them on these medications. Usually, the ob/gyn will suggest an additional method of contraception, such as a condom, to be used with the pill.

Other medications used for narcolepsy include traditional stimulants like methylphenidate (Ritalin), amphetamine salts (Adderall), or lisdexamfetamine (Vyvanse), which are used to help the patient be more awake during the day. Unfortunately, this class of medications tends to have more side effects in terms of heart racing and blood pressure elevation than either modafinil or armodafinil,[6] and they may not be as safe for the long term. If we need to use them, though, we will.

If modafinil or armodafinil don't work, or if they don't work well enough, we may add gamma-hydroxybutyrate (Xyrem), which is what we did with Linda. Gamma-hydroxybutyrate is a very interesting medicine, and it is only distributed by one pharmacy in the United States. It is often referred to as the "date rape" drug,[7] and it results in very deep sleep. As a prescribed medication, it is taken in liquid form just before bed; it helps patients get an extra amount of "delta wave" or N3 sleep, which is restorative sleep (see chapter 2 for more information). We have the patient wake up two and a half to four hours later to take a second dose. This provides another session of very deep sleep, which helps patients feel much better during the daytime.

Since narcolepsy is a disorder of excessive sleepiness, one would think that sufferers must get great sleep at nighttime. But as Linda said earlier, a cruel twist of fate here is that these patients often have disrupted sleep. Coming at it from another direction, narcolepsy can be seen as a disorder of our sleep-wake control system. By that, I mean sleep may intrude on wakefulness (being extremely sleepy or even having a cataplexy attack), and wakefulness may intrude on the sleep period, resulting in insomnia. Treating narcoleptic patients with gamma-hydroxybutyrate can improve the quality of their sleep. Some doctors will put patients on sleeping pills for narcolepsy, with the idea of trying to improve the quality of their sleep, but the mainstay treatment is a stimulant; again, with the intention of pepping them up during the day.

Sometimes, if it's a mild case and the patient doesn't want to take medication, I'll recommend a fifteen- to twenty-minute nap in the middle of the day, plus perhaps coffee. I often will use this approach in pregnant women or those who are nursing (if the coffee is okayed by the patient's ob/gyn), but interestingly, narcolepsy can improve somewhat in pregnancy.

IDIOPATHIC HYPERSOMNIA: EXCESSIVE SLEEPINESS, BUT NO ONE KNOWS WHY

While we're talking about narcolepsy, a disorder of excessive sleepiness, another condition called idiopathic hypersomnia also involves excessive sleepiness. Whenever the term *idiopathic* is used in medicine, it means we don't know exactly why something is happening. *Hypersomnia* means excessive sleepiness. In cases of idiopathic hypersomnia, patients don't have the other features of narcolepsy. The way to know for sure is the PSG/MSLT test discussed earlier. These patients will have the features of sleepiness, but the REM periods seen during naps in narcoleptics will not be present. We can't characterize them as narcoleptics, but we can treat them similarly.

Some people have idiopathic hypersomnia with long sleep times, which means they need as much as twelve hours of sleep per night. Medications may be one answer to the problem. Stimulants (as in narcolepsy) could be the answer. Another could be scheduled naps. Good sleep habits and good sleep hygiene are also important.

Idiopathic hypersomnia can be a frustrating diagnosis for both patients and their doctors. The medications used to treat it may or may not be covered by insurance, and the effectiveness of the medication is often not ideal. Research is currently ongoing in this area of neurology/sleep medicine, and medications with surprising effects such as antibiotics (clarithromycin) may prove useful in the future. A good resource for additional information is the Hypersomnia Foundation's website, http://www.hypersomniafoundation.org/.

FATIGUE: TREAT THE SYMPTOMS AND LOOK OUTSIDE THE BOX

This is a good time to look at the difference between excessive sleepiness and fatigue. They sound like the same thing, but in fact they are not. People who have excessive sleepiness will say that regardless of how much sleep they've gotten the night before, they still could take a nap when they're sedentary. On the other hand, people with fatigue will not report excessive daytime sleepiness; they just don't have the energy to do what they want to do.

While it is possible for someone with a sleep disorder to have both sleepiness and fatigue, the reasons for the two tend to be different. Whereas sleepiness can come from conditions listed previously, from OSA, or from not getting enough sleep in general, fatigue can have more varied reasons. It is harder to pin down the causes, which may include any of the conditions we talked about earlier but also conditions like depression, chronic pain, or fibromyalgia (which is not very well understood). Vitamin deficiencies or certain foods we eat—such as gluten-filled foods—may also be reasons for fatigue. An excellent book on this subject, written by Dr. Mark Hyman, is called the *UltraMind Solution* (2009).

Many patients come to me for fatigue because they are not really sure where to go. We will do a full exam, including a PSG/MSLT and blood work, but in some cases there is no clear answer. In time I suspect we will have a better understanding of what causes fatigue, but for now all we can do is treat the symptoms and try to think outside the box, looking at stress or diet as possible causes.

SUMMARY AND ACTION PLAN

- Narcolepsy and its cousin, idiopathic hypersomnia, are conditions in which excessive daytime sleepiness is the main problem. That is, sufferers have the need to fall asleep in the daytime (even when they do not want to), in spite of how much sleep they have gotten the night before.

- Aside from excessive daytime sleepiness, narcolepsy consists of other symptoms such as cataplexy (which is loss of muscle tone when angry or excited), whereas idiopathic hypersomnia is mostly "just" sleepiness.

- These conditions can only be diagnosed by a sleep specialist, most often after the person in question undergoes an overnight sleep test followed by a nap test (PSG/MSLT). Testing of the blood and spinal fluid can aid in the diagnosis of narcolepsy, but these tests are used much more infrequently than the PSG/MSLT.

- The treatment of these conditions is as follows:

  - Getting enough rest at night is paramount.
  - Short naps (fifteen to twenty minutes) in the middle of the day (time/work permitting) can be very helpful to reduce sleepiness.
  - The most important thing is safety with driving and operating heavy machinery. If the sleepiness in uncontrollable, I advise not driving or operating potentially dangerous machinery until the sleepiness has been properly addressed and treated.
  - Medications that stimulate the body include modafinil, armodafinil, and others such as amphetamines.
  - Gamma hydroxybutyrate (brand name Xyrem) can be extremely effective in narcolepsy, but this is a strange medication that has to be taken at bedtime and again in the middle of the night.

- Fatigue is a little different than excessive sleepiness. Sufferers don't really *fall asleep* in the daytime, but they do not have the energy to do what they want. It can be caused by a variety of health issues and is much more difficult to pin down and treat in many cases.

- Examples of possible causes of fatigue include

  - any of the sleep disorders mentioned in this book
  - conditions like depression, chronic pain, or fibromyalgia
  - vitamin deficiencies
  - certain foods we eat, such as gluten-filled foods

- Bottom line: We don't yet fully understand fatigue, and treatment is basically trying to find and improve the underlying problem.

11

A BROKEN (INTERNAL) CLOCK

Our bodies are controlled by an internal clock that tells us when to sleep and when to wake. This sleep and wake cycle, called our circadian rhythm, is affected by sunlight, temperature, and other environmental clues. When it gets dark outside, we are supposed to fall asleep; when the sun comes out, we are supposed to wake up. But life, as we all know, doesn't always work the way it should.

As a result, many of us suffer circadian rhythm disorders, which include conditions known as advanced sleep phase syndrome, delayed sleep phase syndrome, non-24-hour sleep-wake disorder, shift work disorder, and jet lag.

Any time we talk about circadian rhythms, it is important to mention the impact so-called *blue light* electronic devices—which include televisions, smartphones, tablets, and the like (anything with a backlit display)—can have on our bodies. The blue light these devices emit "tricks" our internal clock into believing that sunlight is coming into our eyes. Sunlight is our most powerful *zeitgeber* (German, for "time giver"), and blue light near bedtime can make our brains think that the sun is out and that we should not be falling asleep. In this situation melatonin is not produced the way it should be and, as a result, it may be hard to fall asleep.

As I said earlier, one of the key factors in sleep hygiene involves shutting off electronic devices that have a backlit screen thirty to sixty minutes before sleep time. Strides have been made recently to reduce the effect of blue light from electronic devices through the development of special blue-blocking glasses (which have an orange tint) and blue-blocking programs and apps. Research about the effectiveness of these measures is still in its infancy, but I think they may be helpful. The best approach, however, would be to just avoid the use of blue light devices before going to bed.

Let's take a look at the disorders of our circadian system.

ADVANCED SLEEP PHASE SYNDROME

In this condition, a person's internal clock has shifted to a point that's earlier than society prefers. Sufferers tend to be elderly people who become sleepy around 6 p.m. to 7 p.m. and are unable to keep themselves awake. They fall asleep, get their seven to eight hours, and then wake for the day at around 3 a.m. They will not usually complain of feeling unrested or other issues, but they are often disheartened because they cannot interact with friends and family the way they would like.

The way to treat advanced sleep phase syndrome is by introducing bright light in the evening, which will delay melatonin production until a more appropriate time. Like many of the remedies I will be discussing in this chapter, it is important to consult with a doctor.

DELAYED SLEEP PHASE SYNDROME

In this condition, which is much more common than advanced sleep phase syndrome, the internal clock is shifted later than society prefers. Delayed sleep phase syndrome (DSPS) tends to occur in teenagers, and a typical scenario would go as follows: A teenager ends the school year and wants to hang out with friends. He stays out until 3 a.m. and sleeps in until he feels ready to get up, as teenagers tend to do. Once school is back in session, the teen's friends are able to realign their internal clock to the required times of going to bed earlier and waking by 7 a.m. or so, but the teen with DSPS cannot.

To treat DSPS, we would urge the person to use bright light in the morning. This can be either an artificial light emitting at least 2,000 lux (a measure of brightness) for twenty minutes or so (not aimed directly at the eyes) or, better yet, getting natural sunlight for twenty minutes. As with advanced sleep phase syndrome, we are using the bright light to shut off melatonin production.

We also use melatonin pills for these people, but it is not the form of melatonin we use for treating insomnia. In circadian rhythm disruption, the dose of melatonin that is recommended is 0.3 mg to 0.5 mg, which is also sometimes written as 300 µg to 500 µg. It is given typically around five hours before the average sleep onset time. It must be taken every night at the same time. For example, let's say someone cannot fall asleep until 4 a.m. In that case, I would have the person take 0.5 mg of melatonin at 11 p.m. every day. This would help, along with bright light in the morning, to readjust their internal clock. If needed, I may also prescribe an actual sleeping pill on top of the melatonin closer to bedtime.

Another therapy, one that has fallen out of favor, is called chronotherapy. The patient is told to go to bed three hours later each night for about one week until their bedtime is matched with what is desired, and then strict adherence to the new schedule is prescribed. This works because it is easier to delay bedtime than to force yourself to get to sleep earlier. Again, this requires close supervision.

An important thing to recognize is that people with circadian rhythm disruption don't necessarily have disrupted sleep. If people with DSPS are allowed to sleep from 3 a.m. to 11 a.m., they will feel fine. Realigning their schedule as much as possible is key. Another way to treat this is by having these patients change jobs or do work that allows for this kind of schedule.

As with all sleep conditions, it makes sense to have a sleep specialist evaluate the situation. The use of sleep logs can help both the doctor and patient examine the sleep schedule at issue. The logs I prefer can be found at the American Academy of Sleep Medicine's website: http://yoursleep.aasmnet.org/pdf/sleepdiary.pdf.

NON-24-HOUR SLEEP-WAKE DISORDER

This is a very rare condition that typically affects people who are blind or are suffering severe psychiatric disturbances. As we discussed earlier, our internal clock is based on cues of light and dark. People who are completely blind may not be able to relate to light in this way. Our internal clock is actually based on a 24.2-hour period of time. This does not seem like a big deal, given that one Earth day is 24 hours. However, with our clock being slightly longer on a day-to-day basis, we have to retrain ourselves with sunlight and darkness. If not, our body's own ability to keep its internal clock at 24.2 hours takes over. Because they cannot use light cues, people who are blind and suffer from non-24-hour sleep-wake disorder eventually become completely out of sync with the 24-hour day.

The way to treat non-24-hour sleep-wake disorder is with medications and regulated sleep-wake schedules. Melatonin, given at consistent times, may be effective. Medications like ramelteon (Rozerem) and tasimelteon (Hetlioz), which are derived from melatonin, have also been shown to be of benefit in this condition.

SHIFT WORK DISORDER

This is a condition that is closely related to a person's work schedule in that there is difficulty sleeping when sleep is desired and there is sleepiness when being wide awake is desired. Other symptoms include poor concentration, fatigue, irritability, depression, and problems with interpersonal relationships.

Not everyone who works shifts suffers from shift work disorder. In those who do, the symptoms can be very difficult to deal with and can result in accidents, mistakes, and other serious issues. The following statistics[1] are from the National Sleep Foundation:

- An estimated 15 percent of the US workforce works outside the traditional nine-to-five workday, which can mean early morning shifts, night shifts, or rotating shifts.
- Approximately 10 percent of night and rotating shift workers are thought to have shift work disorder.
- Between 25 and 30 percent of shift workers experience symptoms of excessive sleepiness or insomnia.

While shift work disorder is a specific condition in and of itself, data suggest that performing shift work on a long-term basis can lead to cancer and other potentially life-altering diseases. The reasons are varied, and while no one theory has been proven correct, it seems that a reduction in melatonin may play a role. The explanation is simple: When shift workers are exposed to light during the night shift, it prevents melatonin from being released into the brain (remember, melatonin is produced when there is darkness at nighttime).

Melatonin, aside from its sleep-wake role, is also a strong antioxidant. Oxidation is a by-product of daily metabolism, and harmful to the body if left unchecked—think of it as a form of inflammation. Melatonin and other antioxidants can help reduce this harmful by-product. Because it reduces melatonin production, working night shifts for a long period of time can lead to increased inflammation. This may result in cancer and other chronic diseases. Compounding this problem further, people who do shift work are often not able to sleep well when they get home, which increases the amount of inflammation the body is exposed to.

Finally, most people who do shift work do not have access to healthy foods. They often rely on vending machines and the like, which is another potential cause for health problems.

To help my patients combat the problems of shift work, I have them take melatonin after the shift is over and when they are in the process of getting home to get to sleep. If they are driving, I may have them wait until they actually get home before they take melatonin. It goes without saying that it is imperative for a shift worker to exercise extreme caution when on the road in a sleep-deprived state, and waiting to take melatonin in this case makes sense.

As soon as they get out of work, night-shift workers should wear sunglasses and try to avoid the sunlight as much as possible. Remember, the sun is our strongest signal that it is time to be awake and to keep melatonin from being produced.

When night-shift workers get home, they should have as dark an environment as possible, using blackout shades or eye masks. Getting quality sleep in the daytime can offset the bad effects of shift work, so daytime sleep becomes even more precious for these people. Sometimes we will use prescription medications to promote sleep.

For work the next day, a good suggestion is to take a thirty-minute nap before the shift begins. Having scheduled naps during the shift would also be helpful, and having bright light before or in the early part of the shift may also help with alertness. We sometimes use stimulant medications such as modafinil (Provigil) or armodafinil (Nuvigil) to help promote wakefulness in these people while they are working. Finally, if the shifts rotate, going forward is ideal. People should try to go to sleep later and later, because going backward is very difficult.

To help us better understand shift work and the problems that can develop in those who undertake it, let's take a look at a real-life example. John, a physician I have known for years, is medical director of an emergency room at a busy hospital in New Jersey. He now mainly works days, but he still puts in two or three overnight shifts per month.

My first real understanding of the value of sleep came during college when I took part in a fundraiser for pediatric cancer that required us to remain awake for forty-eight hours. I drastically underestimated the challenge it would be to my physical well-being, my emotions, and my clarity of thought. Nearing the forty-sixth hour of wakefulness, I had hallucinations and couldn't remember my mother's name. It was almost as if I was drunk.

For a while, I did about six months of hybrid day and night shifts and then, for about two and a half years, I moved exclusively to nights, working from 7 p.m. to 7 a.m. At first, it required a period of adjustment, even though I grew up with a father who worked four nights a week. Any doctor who comes to work in a hospital already has been putting in overnights as part of his or her training, so they understand the basics. But when we hire a technician or somebody who hasn't done this before, I tell the person it's important to plan ahead and see how his or her body reacts to lack of sleep. People need to know how working at night affects their cognition and their happiness.

If you're going to work nights, you should not be a light sleeper because, during the day, you almost certainly will be disturbed and may not be able to get right back to sleep. Whether it's the doorbell ringing, a phone call from a telemarketer, or a neighbor doing construction, you have to be able to get into a deep sleep and ignore distractions.

I now try not to work more than three straight overnights because I know it messes with my body. If I work overnights sporadically, I'll come home in the morning and try to sleep four to five hours. I'll then get up in the mid-afternoon and try to have an active day. That way I'm ready to go to sleep again at the normal hour that night.

Working night shifts takes a lot of preparation. It's taxing. A lot of the women I work with are young mothers who have to go home in the morning to take care of children who don't understand that mom was up all night. They'll get a few hours sleep when the baby's napping, and then they have to go back to work. I honestly don't know how they do it.

The side effects of lack of sleep can be serious. My father had high blood pressure, heart disease, and cancer by the age of sixty-two. His father, who lived to be ninety-two, never had a problem in his life. It's hard to say my father's problems were due to his schedule. On the other hand, he certainly did not have a normal sleep schedule, which has been shown to have remarkable effects on recovery and cardiovascular and neurologic health.

You have to be prepared for the risks of working overnight, which can include detrimental effects on your health and detrimental effects on your family. Overall, working overnights requires a keen sense of self, your sleep needs, your habits, and what fuels your happiness. High-stake jobs often require absolute certainty and clear thinking, which is difficult when you are sleep deprived. Working nights requires the cooperation of family, the understanding of friends, a dedication to recovery time, and an overall commitment to your sense of well-being.

As you can see, shift work can be problematic and shift work disorder can affect anyone. It is therefore important that people who are thinking about shift work as a career should be aware of how a lack of sleep can affect them. Additionally, as John points out, it is imperative to make sure the sleep they get is as efficient as possible.

This section is not meant to scare people who are shift workers. While we know that shift work is not great for our health on a long-term basis, a lot is still unknown. For example, are some people especially vulnerable to the effects of chronic shift work? Are others completely invulnerable? The answers to these and other questions remain to be seen. While it may be difficult or impossible for some people to change their work situations, I advise everyone to consider switching to daytime shifts if they can, and I often write letters on their behalf if that can help.

We tend to underestimate how much a lack of sleep can affect us. But we should never forget instances like the Exxon Valdez oil tanker disaster. The crew had been working through the night and was extremely sleep deprived, a situation that resulted in millions of gallons of oil being spilled into the ocean after the ship crashed into a reef off the coast of Alaska.

JET LAG

Jet lag is basically a process where our internal clock is thrown off after traveling quickly between two or more time zones. Normally, our internal clock is set to the time zone in which we live (our circadian rhythm). It controls not only when we sleep and wake, but also our body temperature and other aspects of our physiology that we don't think about.

When we travel great distances quickly (i.e., on an airplane), our internal clock is often not able to catch up to the local time zone. This was never a problem for our ancestors, or even people living one hundred years ago—they traveled slowly, by foot or horse or boat. These days, traveling through several time zones may result in jet lag.

It can take up to a day for each time zone crossed for the body to adjust, and it is generally more difficult to "catch up" when traveling west to east. During this adjustment period there may be excessive sleepiness or insomnia, along with other symptoms, particularly stomach upset. In older adults, jet lag may hit harder and recovery may take longer.

According to a study reported in the *New England Journal of Medicine*, other factors often aggravate the problem of jet lag.[2] Air cabins pressurized to eight thousand feet may lower oxygen levels in the blood, leading to dehydration and other uncomfortable feelings. The fact that people don't move around as much as usual on an airplane furthers the symptoms of jet lag.

What to do about it? Depending on which direction you are traveling, several things may be useful: If eastbound (the more difficult one), start shifting your bedtime thirty to sixty minutes earlier each night for several nights before leaving. Taking 1 mg to 3 mg of melatonin thirty to sixty minutes before bedtime can help. If you are westbound, the opposite should be done—go to bed thirty to sixty minutes later each night. As discussed earlier, sunlight and bright light help regulate our internal clock. Therefore, when heading east, avoiding early light exposure in the morning and getting as much light as possible in the afternoon and early evening is recommended. Similarly, when heading west, getting bright morning light at the new destination, while avoiding afternoon and evening light exposure, is the way to go.

There are a variety of other simple things to try, most of which involve good sleep habits.

- Try to sleep on the plane if it will be nighttime at the destination upon arrival, or try to stay awake if it will be daytime.
- Moving mealtimes closer to the time of meals at the destination point can be helpful.
- Try to arrive a few days early, so your body can adjust if you need to be on top of your game for an event at your destination
- Drink water before, during, and after the flight to counteract dehydration.
- Avoid alcohol or caffeine a few hours before the desired sleep time; both can disrupt sleep and may cause dehydration.
- Get up and walk around periodically. Do some simple exercises and stretch during the flight. Once at the destination, avoid heavy exercise near bedtime as this can delay sleep.
- Taking melatonin thirty to sixty minutes before bedtime at the destination can help induce sleep. I usually recommend 1 mg to 3 mg.
- A warm bath is always a good thing, and some believe that the drop in body temperature after getting out of the bath may help induce sleepiness.
- Use of an eye mask or earplugs may be useful on the plane and at the destination. Once at the destination, it is advisable to avoid sleep disruptors. Check to make sure that no light is shining in through a window.
- It's usually not necessary to get treatment for jet lag, but sleep medications may help. For those who travel far and frequently, a discussion with a doctor is a good idea.

Here are two free websites that can help you plan for time zone changes when you travel:

http://www.jetlagrooster.com
http://www.timeanddate.com

And a useful article in *Scientific American* on how to prevent jet lag can be found here: https://www.scientificamerican.com/article/how-to-prevent-jet-lag/.

SUMMARY AND ACTION PLAN

Our bodies are controlled by an internal clock that gives us our circadian rhythm and tells us when to go to sleep and when to wake up. Several disorders can affect our circadian rhythm. If you feel that you suffer from any of them, a visit to a doctor is a good idea.

Circadian rhythm problems such as advanced or delayed sleep phase disorders require specific plans to reset the internal clock.

- For those with *advanced sleep phase syndrome*, getting sunlight in the afternoon and doing alerting activities in the early evening can be useful.
- For those with *delayed sleep phase syndrome*, taking melatonin several hours before you plan to sleep, avoiding the use of electronic devices at night, getting sunlight in the morning, and being consistent are all key.
- If you think you have either of these conditions, keeping a sleep log and presenting it to a sleep specialist is a step in the right direction.

Those with *non-24-hour sleep-wake disorder* have an internal clock that is completely out of sync with the 24-hour day. The way to treat this disorder is with medications and regulated sleep-wake schedules. Melatonin, given at consistent times, may be effective, as can medications like ramelteon (Rozerem) and tasimelteon (Hetlioz).

Shift work disorder results in difficulty sleeping when sleep is desired, and sleepiness when being wide awake is desired, as well as other symptoms like poor concentration, fatigue, irritability, depression, and problems with interpersonal relationships. Some ways to combat these issues include:

- Taking melatonin once the shift is over.
- Once out of work, night-shift workers should wear sunglasses and try to avoid the sunlight.

- When you get home, the environment should be as dark as possible.
- Get quality sleep in the daytime.
- Sometimes we use prescription medications to promote sleep.
- Taking a thirty-minute nap before the shift begins.
- Scheduling naps during the shift.
- Getting bright light before or in the early part of the shift may help with alertness.
- Medications like modafinil (Provigil) or armodafinil (Nuvigil) can help promote wakefulness while working.
- If the shifts rotate, going forward (later and later) is better.

Jet lag occurs when our internal clock is thrown off after traveling quickly between two or more time zones. Ways to improve the symptoms include the following:

- If traveling eastbound, start shifting your bedtime thirty to sixty minutes earlier each night for several nights. Melatonin supplements can help. Once you arrive at the destination, avoid light exposure in the morning and try to get as much light as possible in the afternoon and early evening.
- If traveling westbound, go to bed thirty to sixty minutes later each night for several nights. Get bright morning light at the new destination, while avoiding afternoon and evening light exposure.
- There are a variety of other simple things to try, most of which involve the good sleep habits we've talked about.

12

SLEEP AND TECHNOLOGY

While many websites and smartphone apps have been developed to help people track their sleep, I cannot say that I rely on any of them for actual medical decision making. If a patient brings me a readout from one of these devices, I may look at it to see what it says, but I would not utilize it as a basis for making major changes. That said, many of my patients have found sites and apps to be useful and, as I've said throughout this book, as long as it doesn't hurt, it's worth a try. This is going to be a very quick chapter, but the resources listed should be helpful for those interested.

To look at how these technologies can help people to improve their sleep, I'd like to start by referring back to our interview with Audrey in chapter 3. If you recall, her sleep improved after she began to use the Sleep Cycle app. Here are the highlights of a few of the points Audrey shared with us (her interview entries have been slightly edited for brevity and clarity):

> Sleep Cycle is an app I use on my iPhone. You plug into it when you get in bed and it records everything you do during the night.
>
> By journaling my sleep, I became aware of how badly I was sleeping and how many times I was getting up during the night. It was obvious why I didn't feel rested when I woke up in the morning. I'm not sure what kind of algorithms the Sleep Cycle uses, but I could suddenly see the number of cycles of deep sleep I was getting each night, the length of time I was actually in bed, and other things of that nature.

As a result of this new information, I changed my sleep habits. We used to watch TV at eleven o'clock but now we record the news and watch it the next morning while we're getting dressed. I'm in bed before 11 and I usually get up around 6:30. Thanks in part to the app, I'm now getting about seven and a half hours of sleep.

I use the Sleep Cycle app every night, and it tells me exactly when I go to bed, when I wake up and go to the bathroom, and how long I'm up and reading if I can't get back to sleep.

As Audrey's case demonstrates, one of the most useful aspects of these apps (and other technologies) is that they encourage people to become engaged with their sleep and they reinforce, in a way, what I try to do for them. People can look to tracking programs, for example, as a means to monitor their sleep, correlate it with how they feel, or have a more objective sense of how a particular treatment is working for them.

Most of today's sleep-tracking devices, including the ones on smartphones, work by acting as a motion detector. The premise is that someone who is not moving much is asleep, and someone moving a lot is in "light sleep" or awake. In the future, sleep-tracking products may become so fine-tuned that we cannot afford not to use them. For now, I consider them a complement to good medical care at best, and certainly not a substitute.

While many resources exist for those interested in learning more about sleep monitoring, you must be aware that health care and technology are two of the fastest-growing fields, so what is popular and current at the time of the writing of this book (2017) may not be in the near future. As a disclaimer on this subject, I want to point out that I do not have any stake in any of these companies, devices, or publications. The following resources are a good place to start.

For those interested in sleep-related smartphone apps, here are several sites that contain useful information:

- http://www.healthline.com/health/healthy-sleep/top-insomnia-iphone-android-apps#
- http://www.mensfitness.com/life/gearandtech/10-best-mobile-apps-track-your-sleep
- http://www.tomsguide.com/us/pictures-story/679-best-sleep-apps.html

- As a shortcut, simply type the following into a search engine: "healthline insomnia apps," "men's fitness sleep apps," or "tom's guide sleep apps."

A more scientific approach to the subject can be found in a recent comprehensive report published in the *World Journal of Otorhinolaryngology—Head and Neck Surgery*. This article reviews many of the smartphone apps out there,[1] and while it is written with doctors in mind, it is open access and available to anyone who wants to look at it.

The following is a list of wearable technology reviews that I found to be helpful:

- https://www.wareable.com/withings/best-sleep-trackers-and-monitors
- http://www.nosleeplessnights.com/best-sleep-tracker/
- http://gadgetsandwearables.com/2017/03/18/the-best-sleep-trackers/
- Again, as a shortcut, type the following into a search engine: "wearable sleep trackers," "no sleepless nights sleep trackers," or "gadgets and wearables sleep trackers."

Finally, the publication *Sleep Review* has put together a thorough and quite useful analysis of the various online insomnia programs available for purchase;[2] although it is from 2014, the data are still relevant. Some of these programs have specific medical literature to back them up, including SHUTi,[3] CBT-I Coach,[4] Sleepio,[5] and others, which the article summarizes nicely.

SUMMARY AND ACTION PLAN

Many apps and devices are currently on the market, and it is clear that more are on the way. I would summarize my current opinion on them as follows:

- For now, using one of the technologies we talked about in this chapter is not something I feel is necessary.

- They can, however, make you pay more attention to your sleep and your health in general, which is obviously a good thing.
- If you choose to use these apps and technologies, I applaud your efforts to improve your health. As of this writing, however, I don't feel they are precise enough medically to be of great value. But like all things, my guess is that will change in time.

13

DREAMS

There must be a good reason for why we dream. If not, why in the world do we do it?

People often ask me about the significance of dreaming, and, unfortunately, there are no simple answers. A widely held belief is that dreams reflect the concerns a person may have in their wakened life. There are others who think that a dream may impact a person's waking life by offering a source of inspiration, and that therein lies the very purpose of dreams. The bottom line is that no one knows for sure, but it is fun to think and talk about.

Dreaming is part of the bigger question of consciousness—as in what exactly does it mean to be conscious? Most people would say it means we are able to experience the world around us and take in sensory cues, be they visual or sound or touch, and to respond to these cues (emotionally or otherwise).

But can't the same thing be said about a dream?

> We are such stuff as dreams are made on, and our little life is rounded with a sleep.
>
> —William Shakespeare

Think about this: Dr. William C. Dement, who is essentially the founder of sleep medicine, has pointed out in several of his books that when we are asleep, our brain generates not only the content of dreams but also our "sleeping conscious" experience of them. The amount of mental power it takes to perform *both* tasks seems to suggest that dreaming is not some random thing that our brain does just for the hell of it—there must be more to the story.

We talked earlier about the difference between rapid eye movement (REM) sleep and non-REM (NREM) sleep. While it is thought that we dream through the night, the dreams of REM sleep tend to be more action oriented and emotionally charged, whereas in NREM sleep they tend to be more mundane. We have an easier time remembering REM dreams as opposed to those dreams that occur in NREM sleep: When people are woken out of REM sleep, they'll often be able to give a description of what they were dreaming about, a subject many early studies have focused on. Brain areas involved in emotions and memory formation are "reactivated" during REM sleep, which is why there is thought to be an emotional content to dreams, and that memory consolidation is taking place.

Current scientific and psychological studies have told us a great deal about sleep, and in doing so have opened the door to new and exciting theories as to why we dream.[1] Let's go through some of the more interesting ones.

Dreams are often most profound when they seem the most crazy.
—Sigmund Freud

In *The Interpretation of Dreams*, Freud's most famous book, he concluded that some part of our psyche is trying to get out or make itself known through dreams—that dreams are basically ways of wish fulfillment.[2] He hypothesized that we do things in our dreams that we would like to do when we're awake, but we don't because of our inhibitions. Any dream, the theory suggests, no matter how disturbing, can be looked at as a way of getting something you want, in either a literal or symbolic sense.[3]

Some have suggested that dreams are simply internally generated patterns of brain activity during REM sleep, and that dream content does not necessarily have any meaning or message for the individual whatsoever. In other words, this *activation-synthesis theory*[4] puts forth the idea that dreams are an accidental side effect of activated circuits in areas of the brain involved with emotions, sensations, and memories; as the brain attempts to interpret these random signals, the result is dreams.

The *continual-activation theory*[5] of dreaming refers to the idea that our brain is always storing memories, regardless of whether we're awake or asleep. According to this theory, dreams serve as a temporary storage area for memories, as they are moved from short-term to long-term storage. They flash through our minds as dreams before we store them in our "permanent" files, the theory goes.

Yet another possibility is that dreams are based on nonessential information, which is why they tend to have bizarre characteristics to them. In other words, we're essentially filtering out the things from the day that are not important. Dubbed the *reverse learning theory*,[6] this theory suggests that dreams are garbage collection mechanisms, clearing our minds of useless thoughts and making way for better ones.

On the other hand, dreams may help us consolidate our memories. Studies show that people remember what they've learned better if they dream after learning it.[7] In rats, it was found that by going to sleep right after a traumatic experience, the likelihood of remembering the trauma increases for these animals.[8] It has been proposed that one way to help victims of trauma is to actually keep them awake for several hours, even if they are exhausted, to lessen the possibility of them storing the traumatic memory.

Another theory is that dreams prepare us for the stressors of real life; the idea here is that people who experience threatening dreams would be better able to face real threats while awake, presumably because they've already run through these nighttime simulations.[9] Other compelling theories include the thought that dreams act as a type of theater of the mind, during which we are allowed to solve problems,[10] or that dreams allow us to emotionally run through various situations to select the most useful reactions to them.[11]

Finally, the so-called *contemporary theory of dreaming*[12] puts forth the idea that dreaming is a way for the brain to make connections between an emotion felt in a particular situation and a symbol. Thus, those who have experienced trauma (such as an attack or rape) may report a dream of walking on a beach and being swept away by a tidal wave. Dreams, then, are considered to be an evolutionary coping mechanism that helped our ancestors deal with the life-threatening situations and traumas they experienced much more commonly than we do today.

Clinically, figuring out how and why we dream may have applications for mental health in the future. Some have hypothesized that using dreams as a therapeutic approach may be an effective way to deal with certain psychological conditions.

> Dreaming permits each and every one of us to be quietly and safely insane every night of our lives.
> —William C. Dement

As interesting as it is to talk about the theories of why we dream, the scientific study of dreams is unfortunately very difficult to do, as pointed out by Dr. Dement, owing to the fact that to understand the dream world and the thoughts that may be occurring subjectively in the mind requires us to *wake* the person. This will invariably distort the dream, and we're dependent on the dreamer being able not only to remember the dream but also to give us an accurate description of it. But, like many of the situations and conditions we discussed in this book, I am hopeful that we will have a better understanding of dreaming (and sleep) as time goes on.

> Dreams are real while they last. Can we say more of life?
> —Havelock Ellis, British physician and teacher

Switching gears from science to philosophy and religion, let's take a look at what spiritual authorities have said about dreams throughout recorded history. One of the things that got me interested in writing this book is what ancient cultures thought of sleep, particularly dreams. In Ancient Greece and Rome, the predominant view of dreams was that they were divine in origin. This view was held not only in theory but also in practice, as seen by the establishment of various dream oracles and dream interpretation manuals.

Dreams are given special importance in the Bible, both in the Old and New Testaments, as a way in which God or his messengers spoke to man. For example, in the book of Job, it was written, "In a dream . . . when sound sleep falls on men, while they slumber in their beds, then he opens the ears of men, and seals their instruction" (Job 33:16).

In the Book of Acts, the apostle Paul was reassured and was able to provide hope to others through the inspiration given to him in dreams (Acts 16:6–10). And in the Book of Matthew 2:12, the Magi were given instructions to avoid King Herod after meeting with the baby Jesus:

"And having been warned in a dream not to go back to Herod, they returned to their country by another route."

The Jewish patriarchs Abraham, Jacob, and Joseph were inspired by dreams sent by God. In the Talmud, it is stated that dreams can cause distress that will only improve if there is immediate interpretation of the dream. For particularly severe nightmares, it was prescribed that one must fast on the day after the nightmare. The thinking here is that the dream may in fact have been a warning; by fasting and demonstrating repentance, one can reflect and make amends for the issue he or she was being warned about.[13]

The Qur'an, Muslims believe, was information revealed to the prophet Muhammad through the angel Gabriel, from Allah, in the seventh century AD (Qur'an verse 17.106). Sleep is considered by Muslims to be a sign of the greatness of Allah, and they believe that dreams contain a supernatural perception.[14] Muhammad was reported to say, "A good vision is from Allah and a bad dream is from Satan" (Sahih Al-Bukhari 3118).

One Islamic scholar, Al-Qurtubi, who lived in the thirteenth century, considered dreams to be visions seen while the soul is removed from the body during sleep. Nightmares occur when the soul has returned to the body but before it has "taken firm root."[15] The ancient Muslims believed that dreams occurring in the last third of the night contained more truth than others; this is in agreement with our modern knowledge that the last third of the night tends to have more REM (and thus dream) sleep.[16]

In ancient Egypt, the interpretation of dreams, which was the job of the oneiromancer, held that the prophecy of a dream did not mean it would necessarily happen, but that it could happen if the favored treatment—incantation, prayer, and a chemical concoction—had not been completed. One of the most famous prophetic dreams from ancient Egypt was of Thutmose IV, who, around the beginning of the fourteenth century BCE, was reported to have had a dream in which a god spoke to him, inspiring him to restore the Great Sphinx at Gaza; if he did so, he would become pharaoh. This dream was recorded on a plaque between the Sphinx's paws, after he indeed became pharaoh.[17]

The word *rswt*, an ancient Egyptian term for "dream," literally means "to come awake."[18] Some experts have suggested that ancient Egyptians believed that in sleep, one's eyes are open to truths, solutions, or advice. It has been suggested that the ancient Egyptians, particularly those involved in higher learning, were well versed in deeper states of consciousness. Entities called "Mystery Schools" existed, inhabited by "Masters of Secret Things" who were experts in a strange phenomenon known as lucid dreaming. This is a form of dreaming in which the dreamer knows he or she is dreaming, and can somewhat control the content of the dream.

Chinese philosopher Chuang Tzu (300 BCE) once said, "Everything is one; during sleep the soul, undistracted, is absorbed into the unity." In ancient China, dreams were thought to be caused by the dead, whose ghosts required sacrificial offerings for atonement. Others believed the ancestral spirits would attempt to influence the behavior of the living through dreams. Both royalty and common folk felt that dreams bore a religious meaning as well as served as a practical guide for day-to-day life. A major emphasis was placed on honoring one's ancestors, and dreams in which ancestors appeared were seen as having greater importance in terms of religious beliefs and practices.[19]

The ancient Chinese viewed dreams as a spiritual pathway that could aid in understanding the mysteries of life. As an example, Zhuangzi's *Inner Chapters* contains a famous passage: "Long ago, a certain Zhuangzi dreamt he was a butterfly—a butterfly fluttering here and there on a whim, happy and carefree, knowing nothing of Zhuangzi. Then all of a sudden he woke up to find that he was, beyond all doubt, Zhuangzi. Who knows if it was Zhuangzi dreaming a butterfly, or a butterfly dreaming Zhuangzi? Zhuangzi and butterfly: clearly there's a difference. This is called the transformation of things."[20]

It was through this culture that the philosophical tradition of Daoism was founded. One important piece of this philosophy is the concept of yin and yang, which is symbolized by the well-known circle containing black and white elements: yin is the black half with the white dot in it, and yang is the white half with the black dot. The relationship between these is often described in terms of sunlight and a mountain, in which yin represents the shady area darkened by the mountain and yang represents the brightly lit area of a mountain's valley.

This yin and yang philosophy has strong ties to the interplay between wake and sleep, health and illness, and many other aspects of human nature; basically, the concept is that one cannot exist without the other. Given the fact that this is how our processes of wake and sleep operate, the yin and yang symbol has been chosen as the insignia of the American Academy of Sleep Medicine.[21]

The teachings of Socrates, through the writings of Plato, gave us a lot to think about when it comes to our understanding of dreams. For example, Socrates's quote from Plato's dialogue *Crito*: "What evidence could be appealed to, supposing we were asked at this very moment whether we are asleep or awake, dreaming all that passes through our minds or talking to one another in the waking state?"[22] Remember our question of what consciousness *is*? Socrates gets us thinking in this passage, wondering how we can really tell waking life from a dream. It certainly is a thought-provoking question, but one better left for the philosophy books.

Another interesting story about Socrates is that, while awaiting execution, he told of a recurring dream he had had throughout his life. This dream apparently pushed him to pursue the arts, philosophy in particular. Instead of trying to flee his execution, Socrates remained in prison and spent his remaining days translating Aesop's fables into verse; he cited his reason as that he would rather sacrifice his life than betray the guidance given to him through his dreams. Essentially, he wanted to "clear [his] conscience" before taking his "departure."[23] Pretty powerful stuff.

Plato, the student of Socrates, considered dreams to have a divine origin as well as a more bestial source. This passage from his famous work *The Republic* highlights his thoughts: "In all of us, even the most highly respectable, there is a lawless wild beast nature, which peers out in sleep."[24] In essence, dreams, according to Plato, are the time when one expresses the bestial desires that he or she represses in wakefulness.[25]

And of course let's not forget Aristotle, the student of Plato, who, while stating that "nature does nothing in vain,"[26] argued that dreams hold no purpose or function, nor held divine power.[27] They "were the result of persistent sense impressions traveling in the blood stream and activating perceptions in the heart."[28] Aristotle explained away the foretelling of future events based on dreams as mere coincidences. However, he did concede that dreams may be an early sign of medical illness, and thus, in a way, had a role in foretelling the future.[29]

Other major world and religious traditions have had their fair share to say on the always fascinating topic of dreams. For example,

- Some African traditions suggest that dreams are used both for insight as well as treatment of conditions through curative encounters with ancestors and other spiritual entities.[30]
- Native Americans held dreams in high regard, believing that they often played a role in their everyday culture and inspired actions from the design of hunting gear to the specifics of group ceremonies. A special type of dream, called a "Vision Quest," was attained through ritualistic means as a rite of passage and was taken as a source of inspiration and guidance. Similar to the ancient Chinese,[31] Native Americans believed in the existence of two souls—a so-called free soul and a body soul. The free soul is considered to be active while the body is in a passive state, as in dreams, whereas the body soul is bound by different organs.[32]
- In Australian tradition, the Aborigines viewed dreams as a force of creativity provided from the cosmos. They would venture into the process of "Dreamtime" through ritualistic means, or through a vision or a dream itself, and felt that they were engaging with mythic powers when they did.[33]

Lastly, I want to point out the impact that dreams have had on Buddhism and Hinduism; in both orders, dreams were a way of interacting with deities and of foretelling future events.[34] Perhaps the most famous dream in these cultures/religions is that told of Queen Māyā, who was the birth mother of Gautama Buddha, the sage whose teachings later became the foundation for Buddhism. According to legend, during a full-moon night, the queen had a dream in which she felt herself being carried away by four devas (another name for spirits), and was eventually visited by a white elephant. The elephant, holding a white lotus flower in its trunk, entered her womb through her right side. The elephant is a symbol of greatness in India, and the queen realized she had been given a significant message. When she woke, the queen told her husband of the dream, who then had the Brahman priests interpret it. The queen had been childless up to that point, and the priests, based on the dream, predicted that she would bear a son, and that he would either become a great ruler or, if he abandoned his home, he would become a Buddha.[35] As we now know, the latter happened.

Changing time periods one last time, I'd like to close this chapter with a look at what several of our current spiritual authorities have had to say on the subject of sleep. Eckhart Tolle, author of *The Power of Now: A Guide to Spiritual Enlightenment* (1999) and *A New Earth* (2005), placed a strong focus on sleep in his writings. For example, in *The Power of Now*, he makes the claim that when we sleep, especially in deep sleep, our spirit becomes one with the "Source," and through this, we gain energy and vitality for life in the "real" world.[36] To bring us full circle with what we talked about in chapter 2, the deep sleep Tolle is referring to may, in fact, be the N3 (delta wave) sleep that we now know is needed for restoration and energy the next day.

Dr. Wayne Dyer, a contemporary of Tolle's who sadly passed away in 2015, was the esteemed author of many enlightening books, including *Your Erroneous Zones* and *I Can See Clearly Now*. His view of the spiritual aspect of sleep was beautifully stated with this blog entry:[37]

> I choose to impress upon my subconscious mind, and therefore the mind of God to which I am eternally joined, my conception of myself as a Divine creator in alignment with the one mind. . . . I remember that my slumber will be dominated by my last waking concept of myself. I am peaceful, I am content, I am love, I am writing, I am the governing power of the universe, and I attract only to myself those who are in alignment with my highest ideals of myself. This is my nightly ritual, always resisting any temptation to go over any fear or unpleasantness that my ego might be asking me to review. I assume the feeling in my body of those *I am* statements already fulfilled, and I enter my sleep inviting the instruction that my subconscious mind welcomes. I know that I'm allowing myself to be programmed while asleep, for the next day I rise knowing that I am a free agent.

Dyer left us with a great message: thinking positively before going to sleep can be much more beneficial than replaying the bad stuff.

To end this chapter, I would like to point out one last time that dreams are a fascinating part of our reality. That we still do not know much about them makes the understanding and interpretation of dreams one of the last great frontiers for humanity.

CONCLUSION

The concept of why we sleep, and what happens to us when we do, has fascinated man from the beginning of time. As I mentioned at the start of this book, philosophers from Socrates to Plato to Aristotle, from biblical times into the present, have weighed in and contributed various theories and ideas about this intriguing and yet enigmatic subject.

As a neurologist who specializes in treating sleep disorders, I see patients with all forms of sleep problems. Throughout my training and now in my clinical practice, my patients have always been my best teachers. With this book, I have done my best to share what I have learned from them and from the giants of my field, my goal being to help you, the reader, better understand an activity in which you will spend a third of your life.

The importance of sleep can be seen by noticing the effects of its loss on cognition, mood, alertness, and overall health. Many theories have been put forth to explain the function of sleep, including energy conservation, brain and nervous system regeneration, and physical health and performance,[1] but none alone seem to suffice. While this topic has fascinated people throughout the ages, I feel that today we are on the verge of understanding even more fully the nature of why we sleep and what happens to our brain, our body, and mind when we do.

This book was not intended to be a medical text. While it provides clinical advice on the main sleep disorders, it is important, as I have mentioned at many points along the way, to discuss any and all of your medical conditions and sleep problems with your physician.

What I do hope is that this book has deepened your interest in the importance of sleep. I also hope it has shed light on some of the more intriguing aspects of what we know about sleep and what we have yet to uncover.

If you suffer from any sleep disorder, or know someone who does, my hope is that there is enough useful and interesting information here to at least raise awareness of the importance of getting a good night's rest and in some ways begin to address your sleep disorders. It is also my utmost hope that you find as much pleasure and interest in reading this book as I have found writing it.

ACKNOWLEDGMENTS

DANIEL A. BARONE, MD

First of all, I would like to thank God, without whom nothing is possible.

Thank you to Mom and Dad, for showing me unconditional love and support, for believing in me through the years, and for always encouraging me to fearlessly chase after my dreams.

Thank you to my sister, Laura, for being my biggest motivator and supporter, and for always seeing the best in me.

There have been many people on this journey whose help and guidance throughout were invaluable. Thank you PJ Johnson, who urged me to meet up with his writer friend, Larry Armour, to possibly work on a book project. Thank you Larry Armour, for your enthusiasm, patience, and expertise in helping me to turn my dream of writing a book into reality.

I want to thank Joan Parker for your belief in our little team, and for your diligence and efforts to help us get published. Thank you Suzanne Staszak-Silva and all at Rowman & Littlefield Publishing Group for taking a chance on us.

Thank you to my mentors—Drs. Ana Krieger, Avram Gold, Mohammad Amin, Catherine Kier, Rebecca Spiegel, Albert Favate, Paul Mullin, Jay Mancini, Claude Macaluso, Joseph Moreira, Irving Fish, Anthony Geraci, Anne Kleiman, Matthew Ebben, and Howard Sander—for helping me to improve myself and believing in me along the way.

Thank you to those who volunteered to be interviewed for this book. Your time, efforts, and enthusiasm are greatly appreciated. We couldn't have done this without you. And a big thank you to all my patients—as a physician, I have found you to have always been my best teachers.

I would like to express my gratitude to Weill Cornell Medical College, New York–Presbyterian Hospital, the Weill Cornell Center for Sleep Medicine, and all the colleagues and staff members who provide such wonderful service to our patients.

Thank you, Dr. John Rimmer, for being a great friend and for your insight and input to our project. Thank you, Nicholas Zafonte, for your lifelong friendship and contributions to this book. Thank you, Dr. Muhammad Mirza, for your friendship and for taking the time to review the manuscript of this book. Thank you, Christopher Carnaval, for being a loyal friend and for helping me with your contract expertise.

Last, but definitely not least, I want to sincerely thank my friends and loved ones. I would like to give a special mention to the following: Dana Harris, Dr. Joseph Squitieri, Dr. Michael Lodato, Jonathan Bloom, Eric Belanich, Peter Zengota, Phillip Testa, Robert Rennard, Ferdinand Chan, Dr. Kaveh Kashani, Dr. Hind Kettani, Dr. Caroline Geelan, Dr. Zianka Fallil, the Patane and Minuto families, Benjamin Dickerson, Matthew McCarthy, Jared Shellaway, Michael Dunnirvine, Matthew Kabel, and Brendan Burke. Thank you for your support from the bottom of my heart.

> Consult not your fears but your hopes and your dreams. Think not about your frustrations, but about your unfulfilled potential. Concern yourself not with what you tried and failed in, but with what it is still possible for you to do.
> —Pope John XXIII, November 25, 1881–June 3, 1963

LAWRENCE A. ARMOUR

Without being redundant, I'd like to add my thanks to all those on Dr. Barone's list. Your help and support were the key ingredients that made this book work.

I would like to single out Karen Wilder for special thanks. Karen spent untold hours transcribing the interviews on which many of the chapters are based. To say she did a great job under trying circum-stances would be a huge understatement.

Thanks to my wife, Babs, who was there every step of the way, providing the support and encouragement Dr. Barone and I needed. Thanks, too, to my brother-in-law, Dr. Daniel Keller, who made useful suggestions along the way, reviewed the manuscript, and was the link to our hardworking agent, Joan Parker. And thanks, of course, to Dr. Daniel Barone, whose knowledge and insights into all aspects of sleep are amazing, as was the patience he displayed in dealing with my editing.

NOTES

INTRODUCTION

1. J. Bresson, N. Liu, M. Fischler, and A. Bresson. Anesthesia, sleep and death: From mythology to the operating room, *Anesthesia and Analgesia.* 2013; 117 (5):1257–59.

2. A. S. Bahammam. Sleep from an Islamic perspective. *Annals of Thoracic Medicine.* 2011; 6 (4):187–92.

3. S. Ancoli-Israel. "Sleep is not tangible," or what the Hebrew tradition has to say about sleep. *Psychosomatic Medicine.* 2001; 63 (5):778–87.

4. J. Preuss. *Julius Preuss' Biblical and Talmudic Medicine* (New York: Hebrew Publishing Company, 1983).

5. Huangdi. *The Yellow Emperor's Classic of Internal Medicine.* Translated by I. Veith (Berkeley: University of California Press, 2002).

6. N. Ghasemzadeh and A. M. Zafari. A brief journey into the history of the arterial pulse. *Cardiology Research and Practice.* 2011; doi: 10.4061/2011/1648.

7. D. A. Barone, M. R. Ebben, A. Samie, et al. Autonomic dysfunction in isolated rapid eye movement sleep without atonia, *Clinical Neurophysiology.* 2015; 126 (4):731–35.

8. F. Jurysta, J. P. Lanquart, V. Sputaels, et al. The impact of chronic primary insomnia on the heart rate—EEG variability link. *Clinical Neurophysiology.* 2009; 120 (6):1054–60.

9. National Sleep Foundation. Sleep Studies. 2017. https://sleepfoundation.org/sleep-topics/sleep-studies.

10. G. D. Mellinger, M. B. Balter, and E. H. Uhlenhuth. Insomnia and its treatment: Prevalence and correlates. *Archives of General Psychiatry.* 1985; 42 (3):225–32.

11. Y. Chong, C. Fryer, and Q. Gu. Prescription sleep aid use among adults: United States, 2005–2010, *National Center for Health Statistics Data Brief* 127 (2013).

12. Centers for Disease Control and Prevention. 1 in 3 adults don't get enough sleep. 2016. https://www.cdc.gov/media/releases/2016/p0215-enough-sleep.html.

13. Institute of Medicine. *Sleep Disorders and Sleep Deprivation: An Unmet Public Health Problem* (Washington, DC: The National Academies Press, 2006).

I. TROUBLE SLEEPING?

1. M. Hirshkowitz, K. Whiton, S. M. Albert, et al. National Sleep Foundation's updated sleep duration recommendations: Final report. *Sleep Health: Journal of the National Sleep Foundation.* 2015; 1 (4):233–43.

2. A. A. Prather, D. Janicki-Deverts, M. H. Hall, and S. Cohen. Behaviorally assessed sleep and susceptibility to the common cold. *Sleep.* 2015; 38 (9):1353–59.

3. J. Varughese and R. P. Allen. Fatal accidents following changes in daylight savings time: The American experience, *Sleep Medicine* 2001; 2 (1):31–36.

4. S. Abedelmalek, H. Chtourou, A. Aloui, et al. Effect of time of day and partial sleep deprivation on plasma concentrations of IL-6 during a short-term maximal performance, *European Journal of Applied Physiology.* 2013, 113 (1):241–48; K. J. Reid, K. G. Baron, B. Lu, et al. Aerobic exercise improves self-reported sleep and quality of life in older adults with insomnia, *Sleep Medicine* 2010, 11 (9):934–40.

2. THE BRAIN

1. M. Hirshkowitz, K. Whiton, S. M. Albert, et al. National Sleep Foundation's sleep time duration recommendations: Methodology and results summary. *Sleep Health: Journal of the National Sleep Foundation.* 2015; 1 (1):40–43.

2. W. B. Britton, J. R. Lindahl, B. R. Cahn, et al. Awakening is not a metaphor: The effects of Buddhist meditation practices on basic wakefulness. *Annals of the New York Academy of Sciences.* 2014; 1307:64–81.

3. American Academy of Sleep Medicine. *International Classification of Sleep Disorders.* Third edition (ICSD-3) (Darien, IL: American Academy of Sleep Medicine, 2014).

4. A. Rechtschaffen and A. Kales, eds. *A Manual of Standardized Terminology, Techniques and Scoring System for Sleep Stages of Human Subjects* (Washington, DC: United States Government Printing Office, 1968).

5. E. Aserinsky and N. Kleitman. Regularly occurring periods of eye motility, and concomitant phenomena, during sleep. *Science.* 1953; 118 (3062):273–74.

6. S. Banks and D. F. Dinges. Behavioral and physiological consequences of sleep restriction. *Journal of Clinical Sleep Medicine: JCSM.* 2007; 3 (5):519–28.

7. L. Xie, H. Kang, Q. Xu, et al. Sleep drives metabolite clearance from the adult brain. *Science.* 2013; 342 (6156):373–77.

4. INSOMNIA

1. A. J. Spielman, L. S. Caruso, and P. B. Glovinsky. A behavioral perspective on insomnia treatment. *The Psychiatric Clinics of North America.* 1987; 10 (4):541–53.

2. M. D. Mitchell, P. Gehrman, M. Perlis, and C. A. Umscheid. Comparative effectiveness of cognitive behavioral therapy for insomnia: A systematic review. *BMC Family Practice.* 2012; 25 (13):40.

3. L. M. Ritterband, F. P. Thorndike, K. S. Ingersoll, et al. Effect of a web-based cognitive behavior therapy for insomnia intervention with 1-year follow-up: A randomized clinical trial. *Journal of the American Medical Association Psychiatry.* 2017; 74 (1):68–75.

5. DOING WHAT COMES NATURALLY

1. N. Buscemi, B. Vandermeer, N. Hooton, et al. The efficacy and safety of exogenous melatonin for primary sleep disorders: A meta-analysis. *Journal of General Internal Medicine.* 2005; 20 (12):1151–58.

2. A. D. Oxman, S. Flottorp, K. Havelsrud, et al. A televised, web-based randomized trial of an herbal remedy (valerian) for insomnia. *PLoS One.* 2007;

2 (10):e1040; C. M. Morin, U. Koetter, C. Bastien, et al. Valerian-hops combination and diphenhydramine for treating insomnia: A randomized placebo-controlled clinical trial. *Sleep*. 2005, 28 (11):1465–71.

3. National Institutes of Health. State of the science. Conference statement on manifestations and management of chronic insomnia in adults, June 13–15, 2005. *Sleep*. 2005; 28 (9):1049–57.

6. OBSTRUCTIVE SLEEP APNEA

1. T. Young, M. Palta, J. Dempsey, et al. Burden of sleep apnea: Rationale, design, and major findings of the Wisconsin Sleep Cohort study. *WMJ: Official Publication of the State Medical Society of Wisconsin*. 2009, 198 (5):246–49; P. E. Peppard, T. Young, J. H. Barnet, et al. Increased prevalence of sleep-disordered breathing in adults. *American Journal of Epidemiology*. 2013, 177 (9) 9:1006–14.

2. N. C. Wheeler, J. J. Wing, L. M. O'Brien, et al. Expiratory positive airway pressure for sleep apnea after stroke: A randomized, crossover trial. *Journal of Clinical Sleep Medicine: JCSM*. 2016; 12 (9):1233–38.

7. OTHER BREATHING PROBLEMS IN SLEEP

1. R. N. Aurora, S. R. Bista, K. R. Casey, et al. Updated adaptive servo-ventilation recommendations for the 2012 AASM guideline: "The treatment of central sleep apnea syndromes in adults: Practice parameters with an evidence-based literature review and meta-analyses." *Journal of Clinical Sleep Medicine: JCSM*. 2016; 12 (5):757–61.

2. A. R. Gold, F. DiPalo, M. S. Gold, and D. O'Hearn. The symptoms and signs of upper airway resistance syndrome: A link to the functional somatic syndromes. *Chest*. 2003; 123 (1):87–95.

8. MOVIN' IN THE NIGHT, PART I

1. P. Yeh, A. S. Walters, and J. W. Tsuang. Restless legs syndrome: A comprehensive overview on its epidemiology, risk factors, and treatment. *Sleep and Breathing*. 2012; 16 (4):987–1007.

2. S. Mackie and J. W. Winkelman. Restless legs syndrome and psychiatric disorders. *Sleep Medicine Clinics*. 2015; 10 (3):351–57.

3. L. Xiong, J. Montplaisir, A. Desautels, et al. Family study of restless legs syndrome in Quebec, Canada: Clinical characterization of 671 familial cases. *Archives of Neurology*. 2010; 67 (5):617–22.

4. D. L. Picchietti, J. G. Hensley, J. L. Bainbridge, et al. Consensus clinical practice guidelines for the diagnosis and treatment of restless legs syndrome/ Willis-Ekbom disease during pregnancy and lactation. *Sleep Medicine Reviews*. 2015; 22:64–77.

5. N. Silver, R. P. Allen, J. Senerth, and C. J. Early. A 10-year, longitudinal assessment of dopamine agonists and methadone in the treatment of restless legs syndrome. *Sleep Medicine*. 2011; 12 (5):440–44.

6. M. T. Uglane, S. Westad, and B. Backe. Restless legs syndrome in pregnancy is a frequent disorder with a good prognosis. *Acta Obstetricia et Gynecologica Scandinavica*. 2011; 90 (9):1046–48.

7. M. Manconi, J. Ulfberg, K. Berger, et al. When gender matters: Restless legs syndrome. Report of the "RLS and Woman" workshop endorsed by the European RLS Study Group. *Sleep Medicine Reviews*. 2012; 16 (4):297–307.

8. Picchietti, Hensley, Bainbridge, et al. Consensus clinical practice guidelines.

9. J. Montplaisir, S. Boucher, G. Poirier, et al. Clinical, polysomnographic, and genetic characteristics of restless legs syndrome: A study of 133 patients diagnosed with new standard criteria. *Movement Disorders*. 1997; 12 (1):61–65.

10. M. M. Ohayon and T. Roth. Prevalence of restless legs syndrome and periodic limb movement disorder in the general population. *Journal of Psychosomatic Research*. 2002; 53 (1):547–54.

9. MOVIN' IN THE NIGHT, PART II

1. A. Iranzo, A. Fernandez-Arcos, E. Tolosa, et al. Neurodegenerative disorder risk in idiopathic REM sleep behavior disorder: Study in 174 patients. *PLoS*. 2014, 9 (2):e89741; A. Iranzo, J. L. Molinuevo, J. Santamaria, et al. Rapid-eye-movement sleep behaviour disorder as an early marker for a neurodegenerative disorder: A descriptive study. *The Lancet Neurology*. 2006, 5 (7):572–77; R. B. Postuma, J. F. Gagnon, M. Vendette, et al. Quantifying the risk of neurodegenerative disease in idiopathic REM sleep behavior disorder. *Neurology*. 2009, 72 (15):1296–1300; C. H. Schenck, A. L. Callies, and M. W. Mahowald. Increased percentage of slow-wave sleep in REM sleep behavior disorder (RBD): A reanalysis of previously published data from a controlled study of RBD reported in SLEEP. *Sleep*. 2003, 26 (8):1066; C. H. Schenck, B. F. Boeve, and M. W. Mahowald. Delayed emergence of a Parkinsonian disor-

der or dementia in 81% of older men initially diagnosed with idiopathic rapid eye movement sleep behavior disorder: A 16-year update on a previously reported series. *Sleep Medicine*. 2013, 14 (8):744–48.

2. S. P. Lam, S. Y. Fong, C. K. Ho, et al. Parasomnia among psychiatric outpatients: A clinical, epidemiologic, cross-sectional study. *Journal of Clinical Psychiatry*. 2008; 69 (9):1374–82.

3. M. J. Howell. Parasomnias: An updated review. *Neurotherapeutics: The Journal of the American Society for Experimental NeuroTherapeutics*. 2012; 9 (4):753–75.

4. M. J. Howell and C. H. Schenck. Restless nocturnal eating: A common feature of Willis-Ekbom Syndrome (RLS). *Journal of Clinical Sleep Medicine: JCSM*. 2012; 8 (4):413–19.

5. T. I. Morgenthaler and M. H. Silber. Amnestic sleep-related eating disorder associated with zolpidem. *Sleep Medicine*. 2002; 3 (4):323–27.

6. Howell, Parasomnias.

7. C. H. Schenck, I. Arnulf, and M. W. Mahowald. Sleep and sex: What can go wrong? A review of the literature on sleep related disorders and abnormal sexual behaviors and experiences. *Sleep*. 2007; 30 (6):683–702.

8. A. Frese, O. Summ, and S. Evers. Exploding head syndrome: Six new cases and review of the literature. *Cephalalgia*. 2010; 34 (10):823–27.

10. NARCOLEPSY

1. E. Mignot. History of narcolepsy. *Archives Italiennes de Biologie*. 2001; 139 (3):207–20.

2. G. Plazzi. Dante's description of narcolepsy. *Sleep Medicine*. 2013; 14 (11):1221–23.

3. U.S. Xyrem Multicenter Study Group. A randomized, double blind, placebo-controlled multicenter trial comparing the effects of three doses of orally administered sodium oxybate with placebo for the treatment of narcolepsy. *Sleep*. 2002; 25 (1):42–49.

4. T. Verstraeten, C. Cohet, G. Dos Santos, et al. Pandemrix and narcolepsy: A critical appraisal of the observational studies. *Human Vaccines & Immunotherapeutics*. 2016; 12 (1):187–93.

5. Teva Pharmaceuticals. *Provigil (Modafinil): Highlights of Prescribing Information* (North Wales, PA: Teva Pharmaceuticals USA, 1998); Teva Pharmaceuticals. *Nuvigil (Armodafinil): Highlights of Prescribing Information* (North Wales, PA: Teva Pharmaceuticals USA, 2007).

6. T. E. Wilens, P. G. Hammerness, J. Biederman, et al. Blood pressure changes associated with medication treatment of adults with attention-deficit/ hyperactivity disorder. *Journal of Clinical Psychiatry*. 2005; 66 (2):253–59.

7. P. C. Kam and F. F. Yoong. Gamma-hydroxybutyric acid: An emerging recreational drug. *Anaesthesia*. 1998; 53 (12):1195–98; P. E. Mason and W. P. Kerns. Gamma hydroxybutyric acid (GHB) intoxication. *Academic Emergency Medicine*. 2002, 9 (7):730–39.

11. A BROKEN (INTERNAL) CLOCK

1. National Sleep Foundation. Facts about shift work disorder. 2017, https://www.sleepfoundation.org/shift-work/content/facts-about-shift-work-sleep-disorder.

2. J. M. Muhm, P. B. Rock, D. L. McMullin, et al. Effect of aircraft-cabin altitude on passenger discomfort. *New England Journal of Medicine*. 2007; 357 (1):18–27.

12. SLEEP AND TECHNOLOGY

1. A. Ong and M. B. Gillespie. Overview of smartphone applications for sleep analysis. *World Journal of Otorhinolaryngology—Head and Neck Surgery*. 2016; 2 (1):45–49.

2. C. Wolski. 6 online options for insomnia therapy. *Sleep Review*. 2014; December 11. http://www.sleepreviewmag.com/2014/12/online-options-insomnia-therapy/.

3. L. M. Ritterband, F. P. Thorndike, K. S. Ingersoll, et al. Effect of a web-based cognitive behavior therapy for insomnia intervention with 1-year follow-up: A randomized clinical trial. *Journal of the American Medical Association Psychiatry*. 2017; 74 (1):68–75.

4. E. Koffel, E. Kuhn, N. Petsoulis, et al. A randomized controlled pilot study of CBT-I Coach: Feasibility, acceptability, and potential impact of a mobile phone application for patients in cognitive behavioral therapy for insomnia. *Health Informatics Journal*. 2016; June 27.

5. N. S. Coulson, R. Smedley, S. Bostock, et al. The pros and cons of getting engaged in an online social community embedded within digital cognitive behavioral therapy for insomnia: Survey among users. *Journal of Medical Internet Research*. 2016; 18 (4):e88.

13. DREAMS

1. A. Newitz and J. Bennington-Castro. 10 theories that explain why we dream. *Gizmodo.com* (blog), 2013. http://io9.gizmodo.com/10-theories-that-explain-why-we-dream-897195110; M. Schredl. Characteristics and contents of dreams. *International Review of Neurobiology.* 2010, 92:135–54.

2. S. Freud. *The Interpretation of Dreams.* Translated by James Strachey (New York: Basic Books, 2010 [1900]).

3. Newitz and Bennington-Castro. 10 theories; Schredl. Characteristics and contents.

4. J. A. Hobson and R. W. McCarley. The brain as a dream state generator: An activation-synthesis hypothesis of the dream process. *American Journal of Psychiatry.* 1977; 134 (12):1335–48.

5. J. Zhang. Continual-activation theory of dreaming. *Dynamical Psychology.* 2005 (January).

6. F. Crick and G. Mitchison. The function of dream sleep. *Nature.* 1983; 304 (5922):111–14.

7. E. J. Wamsley and R. Stickgold. Dreaming and offline memory processing. *Current Biology.* 2010, 20 (23):R1010–13; E. J. Wamsley, M. Tucker, J. D. Payne, et al. Dreaming of a learning task is associated with enhanced sleep-dependent memory consolidation. *Current Biology.* 2010, 20 (9) 9:850–55.

8. S. Cohen, N. Kozlovsky, M. A. Matar, et al. Post-exposure sleep deprivation facilitates correctly timed interactions between glucocorticoid and adrenergic systems, which attenuate traumatic stress responses. *Neuropsychopharmacology.* 2012; 37 (11):2388–404.

9. A. Revonsuo. The reinterpretation of dreams: An evolutionary hypothesis of the function of dreaming. *Behavioral and Brain Sciences.* 2000; 23 (6):877–901.

10. D. Barrett. "The committee of sleep": A study of dream incubation for problem solving. *Dreaming.* 1992; 3 (2).

11. R. Coutts. Dreams as modifiers and tests of mental schemas: An emotional selection hypothesis. *Psychological Reports.* 2008; 102 (2):561–74.

12. E. Hartmann. The underlying emotion and the dream: Relating dream imagery to the dreamer's underlying emotion can help elucidate the nature of dreaming. *International Review of Neurobiology.* 2010; 92:197–214.

13. S. Ancoli-Israel. "Sleep is not tangible," or what the Hebrew tradition has to say about sleep. *Psychosomatic Medicine.* 2001, 63 (5):778–87; J. J. Askenazy and P. R. Hackett. Sleep and dreams in the Hebrew tradition. In L. Shiyi and S. Inoue, eds. *Sleep: Ancient and Modern* (Shanghai: Shanghai Scientific and Technological Literature Publishing House, 1995), 34–54.

14. A. S. Bahammam. Sleep from an Islamic perspective. *Annals of Thoracic Medicine.* 2011; 6 (4):187–92.

15. Bahammam. Sleep from an Islamic perspective.

16. K. Bulkeley. Reflections on the dream traditions of Islam. *Sleep and Hypnosis.* 2002; 4:4–14.

17. D. Firewolf. The history of dreaming—from ancient Egypt to modern day. *Realmagick.com* (blog), 2011.

18. L. Gillis. And now a word from ancient Egypt. . . . *Dreaminglucid.com* (blog), 2009.

19. C. Pollak, M. J. Thorpy, and J. Yager. *The Encyclopedia of Sleep and Sleep Disorders.* Third edition (New York: Facts on File, Inc., 2009), xvii–xxviii.

20. K. Bulkeley. Dreaming as inspiration: Evidence from religion, philosophy, literature, and film. *International Review of Neurobiology.* 2010, 92; K. Bulkeley. *Dreaming in the World's Religions: A Comparative History* (New York: New York University Press, 2008).

21. Pollak, Thorpy, and Yager. *The Encyclopedia of Sleep and Sleep Disorders.*

22. Plato. "Crito." In E. Hamilton and H. Cairns, eds. *Plato: Collected Dialogues.* (Princeton, NJ: Princeton University Press, 1961).

23. Bulkeley. Dreaming as inspiration.

24. Plato. *The Republic.* In B. Jowett, ed. *The Dialogues of Plato.* Vol. 2. Fourth edition (Oxford: Clarendon Press, 1953).

25. J. Barbera. Sleep and dreaming in Greek and Roman philosophy. *Sleep Medicine.* 2008; 9 (8):906–10.

26. D. Gallop. *Aristotle on Sleep and Dreams* (Warminster, UK: Aris & Phillips, 1996).

27. Heraclitus. *Fragments: A Text and Translation with a Commentary.* Translated by T. M. Robinson (Toronto: University of Toronto Press, 1987).

28. Barbera. Sleep and dreaming in Greek and Roman philosophy.

29. Barbera. Sleep and dreaming in Greek and Roman philosophy.

30. Bulkeley. Dreaming as inspiration.

31. R. K. Ong. *The Interpretation of Dreams in Ancient China* (master of arts thesis). Vancouver, Canada: University of British Columbia; 1981.

32. Firewolf. The history of dreaming.

33. Bulkeley. Dreaming as inspiration.

34. S. Young. Buddhist dream experience. In K. Bulkeley, ed. *Dreams: A Reader on Religious, Cultural and Psychological Dimensions of Dreaming* (New York: Palgrave Macmillan, 2001).

35. Young. Buddhist dream experience. In V. Fausbøll and D. Andersen, *The Jataka: Together with Its Commentary, Being Tales of the Anterior Births of Gotama Buddha*. Vol. 6 (London: Trübner & Co., 1896).

36. E. Tolle. *The Power of Now: A Guide to Spiritual Enlightenment* (Vancouver, BC: Namaste Publishing, 1999), 132.

37. W. Dyer. How do you sleep? *DrWayneDyer.com* (blog). http://www.drwaynedyer.com/blog/how-do-you-sleep/.

CONCLUSION

1. D. A. Barone and A. C. Krieger. The function of sleep. *AIMS Neuroscience*. 2015; 2 (2):71–90.

GLOSSARY

Advanced sleep phase disorder—A disorder of the body's internal clock in which the clock is set too early. For example, someone with advanced sleep phase disorder would prefer going to sleep at 8 p.m. and waking at 4 a.m. Usually seen in older people.

Auto-adjusting positive airway pressure (APAP)—A medical device that uses a varying stream of pressurized air to keep a person's airway open. Used to treat obstructive sleep apnea.

Benzodiazepine medications (sometimes referred to as "benzos")—A medication class that targets the benzodiazepine receptors in the brain. Results in sleep-inducing, antianxiety, and muscle-relaxant properties. Includes Xanax (alprazolam), Klonopin (clonazepam), Ativan (lorazepam), Halcion (triazolam), and Valium (diazepam).

Bi-level positive airway pressure (BPAP, sometimes listed as the brand name, BiPAP)—A medical device that uses two different levels or settings of pressurized air (a "higher" one and a "lower" one) to not only keep an airway open (like continuous positive airway pressure) but also to improve the ability of the lungs to take in oxygen and expel carbon dioxide. Can be used in obstructive sleep apnea, hypoventilation, or hypoxemia.

Blue light—Light in a very special range (around 440 nanometers) that can cause the brain to stop producing melatonin. Many electronic devices with a backlit display emit blue light, including smartphones, computers, TVs, and even some e-readers. Important factor in sleep hygiene and insomnia.

Cataplexy—A symptom of narcolepsy in which there is a loss of muscle tone in the context of strong emotions such as anger or laughter. The loss of muscle tone can be as mild as a weak hand or as profound as a body falling to the ground.

Central nervous system (CNS)—The combination of the brain, spinal cord, and the nerves that travel from them. Responsible for wakefulness, sleep, and all that occurs in each.

Central sleep apnea (CSA)—A disorder consisting of repetitive stoppages of breathing, not due to a blockage of the airway (as in the case of obstructive sleep apnea) but to a failure of the breathing signal coming from the central nervous system. Often seen in cases of congestive heart failure and excessive use of opiate medications, but also for reasons we do not quite understand yet.

Circadian rhythm—The daily cycle of sleep and wake. Essentially, the body's "internal clock." Controlled by the suprachiasmatic nucleus, a special area of the brain that responds to light and darkness.

Cognitive behavioral therapy for insomnia (CBT-I)—A combined treatment approach to improve sleep hygiene and increase the sleep drive. Designed to adjust *behaviors* surrounding sleep, it consists of treatments such as stimulus control therapy and sleep restriction therapy.

Continuous positive airway pressure (CPAP)—A medical device that uses a continuous stream of pressurized air to keep a person's airway open (like an airway splint). Used in the setting of obstructive sleep apnea, usually provided by a home care supplier and paid for by insurance carriers.

Delayed sleep phase syndrome—A disorder of the body's internal clock in which the clock is set too late. For example, someone with delayed sleep phase syndrome would prefer going to sleep at 4 a.m. and waking at 12 p.m. Usually seen in younger people. Typically treated with melatonin and the use of sunlight or bright light in the morning.

Dopamine—A molecule produced in the central nervous system that is used in several facets of brain and body function. Classically, part of the "reward" system that gives pleasure when a particular action is performed or a particular substance is ingested. It plays a major role in addiction and also has a role in sleep and wake. Medications that enhance the functioning of dopamine receptors are used in both Parkinson's disease and restless legs syndrome/periodic limb movements of sleep.

Fatigue—A term for feelings of tiredness that are not necessarily the same as *sleepiness*. Can have many different causes, including sleep problems, depression, vitamin deficiencies, and other problems and conditions.

Ferritin—A measure of the iron stores in the body. When a person has restless legs syndrome (RLS) or periodic limb movements of sleep (PLMS), ferritin levels should be checked. Per the Mayo Clinic, normal ranges are 24–336 in men and 11–307 in women, but in someone who has RLS or PLMS, the range should be above 50–75. Iron replacement pills or iron infusion directly into the blood can raise the ferritin level, as can certain foods. Levels can be low in young, menstruating women. If low in older women or men, a further workup typically needs to be done.

Gabapentin (Neurontin)—A medication that works on the brain and central nervous system to "slow things down." Can be used for headaches, pain, and even epilepsy. Used in the sleep world for insomnia and RLS/PLMS. Closely related to pregabalin (Lyrica).

Gamma-aminobutyric acid (GABA)—A molecule made by the nervous system that "slows things down." Receptors for GABA are located throughout the brain and body, which, when triggered, result in sleep and relaxation. Many medications used in the treatment of sleep-related problems work on the GABA system and can aid in the process of getting to sleep, staying asleep, and treating certain sleep-related conditions such as restless legs syndrome and periodic limb movements of sleep. Gabapentin, pregabalin, zolpidem, and other medications, as well as substances like valerian and alcohol, all have effects on the GABA system.

Gamma-hydroxybutyrate (GHB)—A medication used for narcolepsy that helps the brain achieve very deep sleep. Taken as a liquid, both at bedtime and then in the middle of the night to produce two periods of deep sleep. Only distributed by one central pharmacy in the United States, given its potential for abuse (GHB is the same thing as the date rape drug). Also known as Xyrem.

Glymphatic system—A term for the waste clearance system of the brain. More active and effective during deep sleep, which is one of the reasons healthy sleep is thought to be so important. Without the more effective clearance of deep sleep, waste products build up and over time can result in devastating conditions such as Alzheimer's disease.

Hypnagogic/hypnopompic hallucinations—Either auditory or visual hallucinations that occur as someone is falling asleep (hypnagogic) or waking up (hypnopompic).

Hypnotic—A medical term for sleep-inducing medications and substances.

Hypocretin (Orexin)—A hormone made by the hypothalamus, which controls wakefulness. When it is deficient, narcolepsy results.

Hypoglossal nerve—The nerve that controls the tongue muscle.

Hypoglossal nerve stimulation—A surgical procedure in which an electric stimulator is implanted in a person's chest and wired to the hypoglossal nerve. When activated, the stimulator causes the nerve to tell the tongue muscle to stiffen, which lessens the possibility of the tongue falling to the back of the throat as in the case of obstructive sleep apnea.

Hypothalamus—A structure that sits in the brain and controls many of the things we do not think about. Hunger, temperature, and sleep and wake are controlled by the hormones made in the hypothalamus.

Hypoventilation—A condition that occurs when the lungs are unable to get rid of the carbon dioxide in the blood (sometimes referred to as respiratory depression). Causes include neurologic illness (like Lou Gehrig's disease), certain medications or illicit drugs (like opioid or benzodiazepine medications when taken in excess), and obesity (a condition known as obesity-hypoventilation syndrome). Treated with bilevel positive airway pressure (BPAP, also known as the brand name BiPAP).

Hypoxemia—Low oxygen in the blood, the result of a lack of effectiveness of the lungs. Caused by chronic obstructive pulmonary disease (COPD), severe asthma, obesity, neurologic illness, sleep apnea (both obstructive and central), and very high altitude. Treatment may include the use of supplemental oxygen (as in COPD), weight loss (sometimes bariatric surgery), continuous positive airway pressure (CPAP), bi-level positive airway pressure (BPAP, also known as the brand name BiPAP), or variable positive airway pressure (VPAP, also known as adaptive servo ventilation, ASV).

Idiopathic hypersomnia—A condition in which there is chronic excessive daytime sleepiness that does not have the other features of narcolepsy (cataplexy, sleep paralysis, and hypnagogic/hypnopompic hallucinations). Diagnosed through a combination of an overnight sleep test (polysomnogram) plus a next-day nap test (multiple sleep latency test). Called idiopathic because it is not known (at this time) why it occurs.

Jet lag—A benign condition that occurs when traveling through several time zones. Results in feeling the need to sleep when it is the middle of the day, and feeling wide awake when it is the middle of the night. Other symptoms may include upset stomach or headaches.

Mandibular advancement device (MAD)—A medical appliance that sits over both the upper and lower sets of teeth. Used to "pull" the lower jaw (the mandible) forward a few millimeters when worn at bedtime. The MAD pulls the tongue and soft tissues away from the back of the throat and opens the upper airway. Used to treat snoring and obstructive sleep apnea. While a high-quality version is usually made by a dentist (useful for obstructive sleep apnea), a temporary one can be purchased online (useful for snoring).

Melatonin—A hormone, made by the pineal gland, which regulates our internal clock. Produced normally when the sun goes down but can be prevented from being released by "blue light" devices. Can be taken in pill or liquid form to help with insomnia and other sleep disturbances.

Multiple sleep latency test (MSLT)—A nap test used to determine a person's level of sleepiness. Useful in the diagnosis of narcolepsy and idiopathic hypersomnia.

Narcolepsy—A somewhat rare condition in which there is excessive daytime sleepiness due to a lack of a hormone (hypocretin, orexin) being produced in the brain. The condition includes other symptoms such as cataplexy (loss of muscle control usually seen in the context of laughter or anger), sleep paralysis, and hypnagogic/hypnopompic hallucinations.

Non-benzodiazepine medications (the "non-benzos," also known as the "Z" drugs)—A medication class that has some effects similar to the benzo drugs, particularly the sleep-inducing properties but without the antianxiety and muscle relaxation properties. Examples include Lunesta (eszopiclone), Ambien (zolpidem), and Sonata (zaleplon).

Non–rapid eye movement sleep (NREM sleep)—A form of sleep that is different from rapid eye movement, or REM, sleep in that there is no paralysis of the muscles, and while dreams can occur, they are much less emotional and action packed. The majority of sleep time is spent in NREM sleep. There are three stages, conveniently labeled N1 (the lightest), N2 (the baseline), and N3 (very deep).

Obstructive sleep apnea (OSA)—A common disorder in which there are repetitive stoppages of breathing while someone is asleep. Usually due to the tongue and/or soft tissues falling toward the back of the throat. Sometimes referred to simply as sleep apnea.

Parasomnia—An abnormal movement or sensation that occurs close to sleep onset or during the night. Sleepwalking is a good example of an abnormal movement, while hypnagogic or hypnopompic hallucinations are good examples of abnormal sensations.

Periodic limb movements of sleep (PLMS)—A condition often seen with restless legs syndrome. The legs (and sometimes the arms) move throughout the night, potentially disrupting sleep (in which case it is known as periodic limb movement disorder, PLMD).

Pineal gland—An area of the brain once thought to be "the seat of the soul." Sits in the middle of the brain and produces melatonin when activated by the suprachiasmatic nucleus.

Polysomnography—An overnight sleep test during which electrodes, wires, and belts are placed on multiple areas of a patient's body, including the scalp, to obtain objective information about how the patient sleeps. It is the basis for the diagnosis of obstructive sleep apnea, periodic limb movements of sleep, parasomnias, and several other disorders.

Positive airway pressure (PAP)—A medical technology that involves the use of a device to create pressurized air, which in turn is applied to the nose or mouth through a mask to keep a person's airway open (like an airway splint). Various forms include continuous positive airway pressure (CPAP), bi-level positive airway pressure (BPAP, also known as the brand name, BiPAP), variable positive airway pressure (VPAP, also known as adaptive servo ventilation, ASV), and auto-adjusting positive airway pressure (APAP). All forms utilize a small machine; a six-foot-long tube; and either a nasal pillow interface, a nasal mask, or a full-face mask.

Rapid eye movement sleep (REM sleep)—A form of sleep in which the eyes move rapidly (hence the name) while a person is otherwise paralyzed. Sometimes referred to as "dream sleep." During a normal night of sleep, 20–25 percent of the time is spent in REM, broken into four or five periods over the course of the night.

REM behavior disorder (RBD)—A condition in which the muscle paralysis that normally occurs in REM sleep no longer happens. Sufferers will often act out their dreams and can hurt themselves or others.

Restless legs syndrome (RLS)—A common condition in which uncomfortable sensations in the legs (and sometimes the arms) result in difficulty falling asleep. Often seen with periodic limb movements of sleep. The four main symptoms, known by the acronym "URGE," consist of U for the urge to move, R for a feeling of restlessness, G for go (when the sufferer gets up and goes, the symptoms resolve), and E for evening (which is when the symptoms become problematic).

Shift work disorder—A condition affecting people who work either rotating shifts or night shifts. Consists of excessive sleepiness when it is necessary to be alert, and insomnia when sleep is needed.

Sleep cycles—A period of time within a normal night of sleep in which the brain travels through the various stages and usually ends with a period of REM sleep. Lasts approximately 90 minutes, with four or five cycles occurring over the course of a normal sleep period.

Sleep drive—A signal from the brain's sleep "thermostat." In a normal situation, if people have been awake for sixteen hours, their sleep thermostat will tell them they are tired and need to sleep. This is called sleep drive or the drive to sleep. Some cognitive behavioral therapy approaches are effective because they increase sleep drive, making sleep easier to achieve.

Sleep hygiene—A collection of practices that aid in healthy sleep when done correctly. If sleep hygiene is poor, it can impede the ability to sleep. Improving sleep hygiene is essential in the treatment of chronic insomnia.

Sleep paralysis—A strange phenomenon in which someone is physically unable to move, either as they are falling asleep or waking up. It can happen in conjunction with hallucinations. Most people experience sleep paralysis on rare occasions, in which case it is benign. If it occurs more frequently, it can be a sign of certain sleep disorders, narcolepsy in particular.

Sleep starts—A benign condition consisting of sudden, brief, and strong contractions of the body that occur as someone is falling asleep. May be accompanied by a scream or a sensation of falling or tripping. Sleep starts happen more frequently in cases where there is excess caffeine, high stress, vigorous exercise, poor sleep, or not enough sleep. Also known as hypnic jerks.

Snoring—A very common condition that occurs when the upper airway is at least partially blocked off and vibratory sounds are produced. Can be seen in cases of obstructive sleep apnea, but not all sufferers of obstructive sleep apnea snore, and vice versa. Usually worsened by sleeping on the back or drinking alcohol.

Soft palate—The soft, flexible portion of the roof of the mouth, located behind the hard palate. Along with the uvula, can produce snoring when it vibrates. Can be shaven down to reduce snoring (and sometimes obstructive sleep apnea) during a procedure called an uvulopalatopharyngoplasty.

Stimulant medications—Classes of medications used to treat excessive daytime sleepiness. Includes non-amphetamines such as Provigil (modafinil), Nuvigil (armodafinil), Ritalin/Concerta (methylphenidate), and Focalin (dexmethylphenidate). Amphetamine-based stimulants include Adderall (amphetamine/dextroamphetamine) and Vyvanse (lisdexamfetamine).

Suprachiasmatic nucleus (SCN)—An area of the brain that sits directly above the nerves coming to and from the eyes. When the sun goes down, the suprachiasmatic nucleus activates the pineal gland to produce melatonin.

Suvorexant (Belsomra)—A newer medication for insomnia that works by blocking the wake signal of the brain (as opposed to enhancing the sleep signals, which all other hypnotics do).

Upper airway—Consists of the nose, the mouth, the tongue, and other soft tissues such as tonsils and the uvula. These structures vibrate in the case of snoring, and lead to obstructions in the case of obstructive sleep apnea.

Upper airway resistance syndrome (UARS)—A form of a "tight" airway that is not as blocked off as in obstructive sleep apnea. Although symptoms may be different from obstructive sleep apnea and include fatigue and other problems, the treatment is the same as it is with OSA.

Uvula—A piece of tissue that hangs in the back of the throat and looks like a "punching bag." Mainly used for producing certain sounds but is essentially not needed in the human body. When the uvula vibrates rapidly it produces snoring, and when removed surgically it can improve snoring. Often removed for snoring in a procedure known as an uvulopalatopharyngoplasty.

Uvulopalatopharyngoplasty (UPPP)—A surgical procedure in which the uvula as well as parts of the soft palate are removed from the back of the throat. Viewed as a possible treatment for obstructive sleep apnea, but mostly improves snoring.

Variable positive airway pressure (VPAP, also known as adaptive servo ventilation, ASV)—A medical device that uses multiple levels or settings of pressurized air to keep an airway open (like continuous positive airway pressure). Also used to improve the ability of the lungs to take in oxygen and expel carbon dioxide (like bi-level positive airway pressure) and to essentially "breathe" for the patient in cases of central sleep apnea. Can be used to treat obstructive sleep apnea, hypoventilation or hypoxemia, or central sleep apnea.

BIBLIOGRAPHY AND ADDITIONAL RESOURCES

BIBLIOGRAPHY BY CHAPTER

Introduction

Ancoli-Israel, S. "Sleep is not tangible," or what the Hebrew tradition has to say about sleep. *Psychosomatic Medicine.* 2001; 63 (5):778–87.

Bahammam, A. S. Sleep from an Islamic perspective. *Annals of Thoracic Medicine.* 2011; 6 (4):187–92.

Barone, D. A., M. R. Ebben, A. Samie, et al. Autonomic dysfunction in isolated rapid eye movement sleep without atonia. *Clinical Neurophysiology.* 2015; 126 (4):731–35.

Bresson, J., N. Liu, M. Fischler, and A. Bresson. Anesthesia, sleep and death: From mythology to the operating room. *Anesthesia and Analgesia.* 2013; 117 (5):1257–59.

Centers for Disease Control and Prevention. 1 in 3 adults don't get enough sleep. 2016, https://www.cdc.gov/media/releases/2016/p0215-enough-sleep.html.

Chong, Y., C. Fryer, and Q. Gu. Prescription sleep aid use among adults: United States, 2005–2010. *National Center for Health Statistics Data Brief.* 2013; 127.

Ghasemzadeh, N., and A. M. Zafari. A brief journey into the history of the arterial pulse. *Cardiology Research and Practice.* 2011. doi: 10.4061/2011/164832.

Huangdi. *The Yellow Emperor's Classic of Internal Medicine.* Translated by I. Veith. Berkeley: University of California Press, 2002.

Institute of Medicine. *Sleep Disorders and Sleep Deprivation: An Unmet Public Health Problem.* Washington, DC: The National Academies Press, 2006.

Jurysta, F., J. P. Lanquart, V. Sputaels, et al. The impact of chronic primary insomnia on the heart rate—EEG variability link. *Clinical Neurophysiology.* 2009; 120 (6):1054–60.

Mellinger, G. D., M. B. Balter, and E. H. Uhlenhuth. Insomnia and its treatment. Prevalence and correlates. *Archives of General Psychiatry.* 1985; 42 (3):225–32.

National Sleep Foundation. Sleep Studies. 2017. https://sleepfoundation.org/sleep-topics/sleep-studies.

Preuss, J. *Julius Preuss' Biblical and Talmudic Medicine.* New York: Hebrew Publishing Company, 1983.

Chapter 1

Abedelmalek, S., H. Chtourou, A. Aloui, et al. Effect of time of day and partial sleep deprivation on plasma concentrations of IL-6 during a short-term maximal performance. *European Journal of Applied Physiology*. 2013; 113 (1):241–48.

Hirshkowitz, M., K. Whiton, S. M. Albert, et al. National Sleep Foundation's updated sleep duration recommendations: Final report. *Sleep Health: Journal of the National Sleep Foundation*. 2015; 1 (4):233–43.

Prather, A. A., D. Janicki-Deverts, M. H. Hall, and S. Cohen. Behaviorally assessed sleep and susceptibility to the common cold. *Sleep*. 2015; 38 (9):1353–59.

Reid, K. J., K. G. Baron, B. Lu, et al. Aerobic exercise improves self-reported sleep and quality of life in older adults with insomnia. *Sleep Medicine*. 2010; 11 (9):934–40.

Varughese, J., and R. P. Allen. Fatal accidents following changes in daylight savings time: The American experience. *Sleep Medicine*. 2001; 2 (1):31–36.

Chapter 2

American Academy of Sleep Medicine. *International Classification of Sleep Disorders*. Third edition (ICSD-3). Darien, IL: American Academy of Sleep Medicine, 2014.

Aserinsky, E., and N. Kleitman. Regularly occurring periods of eye motility, and concomitant phenomena, during sleep. *Science*. 1953; 118 (3062):273–74.

Banks, S., and D. F. Dinges. Behavioral and physiological consequences of sleep restriction. *Journal of Clinical Sleep Medicine: JCSM*. 2007; 3 (5):519–28.

Britton, W. B., J. R. Lindahl, B. R. Cahn, et al. Awakening is not a metaphor: The effects of Buddhist meditation practices on basic wakefulness. *Annals of the New York Academy of Sciences*. 2014; 1307:64–81.

Hirshkowitz, M., K. Whiton, S. M. Albert, et al. National Sleep Foundation's sleep time duration recommendations: Methodology and results summary. *Sleep Health: Journal of the National Sleep Foundation*. 2015; 1 (1):40–43.

Rechtschaffen, A., and A. Kales, eds. *A Manual of Standardized Terminology, Techniques and Scoring System for Sleep Stages of Human Subjects*. Washington, DC: United States Government Printing Office, 1968.

Xie, L., H. Kang, Q. Xu, et al. Sleep drives metabolite clearance from the adult brain. *Science*. 2013; 342 (6156):373–77.

Chapter 4

Mitchell, M. D., P. Gehrman, M. Perlis, and C. A. Umscheid. Comparative effectiveness of cognitive behavioral therapy for insomnia: A systematic review. *BMC Family Practice*. 2012; 25 (13):40.

Ritterband, L. M., F. P. Thorndike, K. S. Ingersoll, et al. Effect of a web-based cognitive behavior therapy for insomnia intervention with 1-year follow-up: A randomized clinical trial. *Journal of the American Medical Association Psychiatry*. 2017; 74 (1):68–75.

Spielman, A. J., L. S. Caruso, and P. B. Glovinsky. A behavioral perspective on insomnia treatment. *Psychiatric Clinics of North America*. 1987; 10 (4):541–53.

Chapter 5

Buscemi, N., B. Vandermeer, N. Hooton, et al. The efficacy and safety of exogenous melatonin for primary sleep disorders: A meta-analysis. *Journal of General Internal Medicine*. 2005; 20 (12):1151–58.

Morin, C. M., U. Koetter, C. Bastien, et al. Valerian-hops combination and diphenhydramine for treating insomnia: A randomized placebo-controlled clinical trial. *Sleep*. 2005; 28 (11):1465–71.
National Institutes of Health. State of the science. Conference statement on manifestations and management of chronic insomnia in adults, June 13–15, 2005. *Sleep*. 2005; 28 (9):1049–57.
Oxman, A. D., S. Flottorp, K. Havelsrud, et al. A televised, web-based randomized trial of an herbal remedy (valerian) for insomnia. *PLoS One*. 2007; 2 (10):e1040.

Chapter 6

Peppard, P. E., T. Young, J. H. Barnet, et al. Increased prevalence of sleep-disordered breathing in adults. *American Journal of Epidemiology*. 2013; 177 (9):1006–14.
Wheeler, N. C., J. J. Wing, L. M. O'Brien, et al. Expiratory positive airway pressure for sleep apnea after stroke: A randomized, crossover trial. *Journal of Clinical Sleep Medicine: JCSM*. 2016; 12 (9):1233–38.
Young, T., M. Palta, J. Dempsey, et al. Burden of sleep apnea: Rationale, design, and major findings of the Wisconsin Sleep Cohort study. *WMJ: Official Publication of the State Medical Society of Wisconsin*. 2009; 198 (5):246–49.

Chapter 7

Aurora, R. N., S. R. Bista, K. R. Casey, et al. Updated adaptive servo-ventilation recommendations for the 2012 AASM guideline: "The treatment of central sleep apnea syndromes in adults: Practice parameters with an evidence-based literature review and meta-analyses." *Journal of Clinical Sleep Medicine: JCSM*. 2016; 12 (5):757–61.
Gold, A. R., F. DiPalo, M. S. Gold, and D. O'Hearn. The symptoms and signs of upper airway resistance syndrome: A link to the functional somatic syndromes. *Chest*. 2003; 123 (1):87–95.

Chapter 8

Mackie, S., and J. W. Winkelman. Restless legs syndrome and psychiatric disorders. *Sleep Medicine Clinics*. 2015; 10 (3):351–57.
Manconi, M., J. Ulfberg, K. Berger, et al. When gender matters: Restless legs syndrome. Report of the "RLS and woman" workshop endorsed by the European RLS Study Group. *Sleep Medicine Reviews*. 2012; 16 (4):297–307.
Montplaisir, J., S. Boucher, G. Poirier, et al. Clinical, polysomnographic, and genetic characteristics of restless legs syndrome: A study of 133 patients diagnosed with new standard criteria. *Movement Disorders*. 1997; 12 (1):61–65.
Ohayon, M. M., and T. Roth. Prevalence of restless legs syndrome and periodic limb movement disorder in the general population. *Journal of Psychosomatic Research*. 2002; 53 (1):547–54.
Picchietti, D. L., J. G. Hensley, J. L. Bainbridge, et al. Consensus clinical practice guidelines for the diagnosis and treatment of restless legs syndrome/Willis-Ekbom disease during pregnancy and lactation. *Sleep Medicine Reviews*. 2015; 22:64–77.
Silver, N., R. P. Allen, J. Senerth, and C. J. Early. A 10-year, longitudinal assessment of dopamine agonists and methadone in the treatment of restless legs syndrome. *Sleep Medicine*. 2011; 12 (5):440–44.

Uglane, M. T., S. Westad, and B. Backe. Restless legs syndrome in pregnancy is a frequent disorder with a good prognosis. *Acta Obstetricia et Gynecologica Scandinavica.* 2011; 90 (9):1046–48.

Xiong, L., J. Montplaisir, A. Desautels, et al. Family study of restless legs syndrome in Quebec, Canada: Clinical characterization of 671 familial cases. *Archives of Neurology.* 2010; 67 (5):617–22.

Yeh, P., A. S. Walters, and J. W. Tsuang. Restless legs syndrome: A comprehensive overview on its epidemiology, risk factors, and treatment. *Sleep and Breathing.* 2012; 16 (4):987–1007.

Chapter 9

Frese, A., O. Summ, and S. Evers. Exploding head syndrome: Six new cases and review of the literature. *Cephalalgia.* 2014; 34 (10):823–27.

Howell, M. J. Parasomnias: An updated review. *Neurotherapeutics.* 2012; 9 (4):753–75.

Howell, M. J., and C. H. Schenck. Restless nocturnal eating: A common feature of Willis-Ekbom Syndrome (RLS). *Journal of Clinical Sleep Medicine: JCSM.* 2012; 8 (4):413–19.

Iranzo, A., A. Fernandez-Arcos, E. Tolosa, et al. Neurodegenerative disorder risk in idiopathic REM sleep behavior disorder: Study in 174 patients. *PLoS.* 2014; 9 (2):e89741.

Iranzo, A., J. L. Molinuevo, J. Santamaria, et al. Rapid-eye-movement sleep behaviour disorder as an early marker for a neurodegenerative disorder: A descriptive study. *Lancet Neurology.* 2006; 5 (7):572–77.

Lam, S. P., S. Y. Fong, C. K. Ho, et al. Parasomnia among psychiatric outpatients: A clinical, epidemiologic, cross-sectional study. *Journal of Clinical Psychiatry.* 2008; 69 (9):1374–82.

Morgenthaler, T. I., and M. H. Silber. Amnestic sleep-related eating disorder associated with zolpidem. *Sleep Medicine.* 2002; 3 (4):323–27.

Postuma, R. B., J. F. Gagnon, M. Vendette, et al. Quantifying the risk of neurodegenerative disease in idiopathic REM sleep behavior disorder. *Neurology.* 2009; 72 (15):1296–300.

Schenck, C. H., I. Arnulf, and M. W. Mahowald. Sleep and sex: What can go wrong? A review of the literature on sleep related disorders and abnormal sexual behaviors and experiences. *Sleep.* 2007; 30 (6):683–702.

Schenck, C. H., B. F. Boeve, and M. W. Mahowald. Delayed emergence of a Parkinsonian disorder or dementia in 81% of older men initially diagnosed with idiopathic rapid eye movement sleep behavior disorder: A 16-year update on a previously reported series. *Sleep Medicine.* 2013; 14 (8):744–48.

Schenck, C. H., A. L. Callies, and M. W. Mahowald. Increased percentage of slow-wave sleep in REM sleep behavior disorder (RBD): A reanalysis of previously published data from a controlled study of RBD reported in SLEEP. *Sleep.* 2003; 26 (8):1066.

Chapter 10

Kam, P. C., and F. F. Yoong. Gamma-hydroxybutyric acid: An emerging recreational drug. *Anaesthesia.* 1998; 53 (12):1195–98.

Mason, P. E., and W. P. Kerns. Gamma hydroxybutyric acid (GHB) intoxication. *Academic Emergency Medicine.* 2002; 9 (7):730–39.

Mignot, E. History of narcolepsy. *Archives Italiennes de Biologie.* 2001; 139 (3):207–20.

Plazzi, G. Dante's description of narcolepsy. *Sleep Medicine.* 2013; 14 (11):1221–23.

Teva Pharmaceuticals. *Nuvigil (Armodafinil): Highlights of prescribing information.* North Wales, PA: Teva Pharmaceuticals USA, 2007.

Teva Pharmaceuticals. *Provigil (Modafinil): Highlights of prescribing information.* North Wales, PA: Teva Pharmaceuticals USA, 1998.

U.S. Xyrem Multicenter Study Group. A randomized, double blind, placebo-controlled multicenter trial comparing the effects of three doses of orally administered sodium oxybate with placebo for the treatment of narcolepsy. *Sleep*. 2002; 25 (1):42–49.

Verstraeten, T., C. Cohet, G. Dos Santos, et al. Pandemrix and narcolepsy: A critical appraisal of the observational studies. *Human Vaccines & Immunotherapeutics*. 2016; 12 (1):187–93.

Wilens, T. E., P. G. Hammerness, J. Biederman, et al. Blood pressure changes associated with medication treatment of adults with attention-deficit/hyperactivity disorder. *Journal of Clinical Psychiatry*. 2005; 66 (2):253–59.

Chapter 11

Muhm, J. M., P. B. Rock, D. L. McMullin, et al. Effect of aircraft-cabin altitude on passenger discomfort. *New England Journal of Medicine*. 2007; 357 (1):18–27.

National Sleep Foundation. Facts about shift work disorder. 2017. https://www.sleepfoundation.org/shift-work/content/facts-about-shift-work-sleep-disorder.

Chapter 12

Coulson, N. S., R. Smedley, S. Bostock, et al. The pros and cons of getting engaged in an online social community embedded within digital cognitive behavioral therapy for insomnia: Survey among users. *Journal of Medical Internet Research*. 2016; 18 (4):e88.

Koffel, E., E. Kuhn, N. Petsoulis, et al. A randomized controlled pilot study of CBT-I Coach: Feasibility, acceptability, and potential impact of a mobile phone application for patients in cognitive behavioral therapy for insomnia. *Health Informatics Journal*. 2016; June 27.

Ong, A., and M. B. Gillespie. Overview of smartphone applications for sleep analysis. *World Journal of Otorhinolaryngology-Head and Neck Surgery*. 2016; 2 (1):45–49.

Ritterband, L. M., F. P. Thorndike, K. S. Ingersoll, et al. Effect of a web-based cognitive behavior therapy for insomnia intervention with 1-year follow-up: A randomized clinical trial. *Journal of the American Medical Association Psychiatry*. 2017; 74 (1):68–75.

Wolski, C. 6 online options for insomnia therapy, *Sleep Review*. 2014; December 11. http://www.sleepreviewmag.com/2014/12/online-options-insomnia-therapy/.

Chapter 13

Ancoli-Israel, S. "Sleep is not tangible," or what the Hebrew tradition has to say about sleep. *Psychosomatic Medicine*. 2001; 63 (5):778–87.

Askenazy, J. J., and P. R. Hackett. Sleep and dreams in the Hebrew tradition. In L. Shiyi and S. Inoue, eds. *Sleep: Ancient and Modern*, 34–54. Shanghai: Shanghai Scientific and Technological Literature Publishing House, 1995.

Bahammam, A. S. Sleep from an Islamic perspective. *Annals of Thoracic Medicine*. 2011; 6 (4):187–92.

Barbera, J. Sleep and dreaming in Greek and Roman philosophy. *Sleep Medicine*. 2008; 9 (8):906–10.

Barrett, D. "The committee of sleep": A study of dream incubation for problem solving. *Dreaming*. 1993; 3 (2).

Bulkeley, K. Dreaming as inspiration: Evidence from religion, philosophy, literature, and film. *International Review of Neurobiology*. 2010; 92.

Bulkeley, K. *Dreaming in the World's Religions: A Comparative History*. New York: New York University Press, 2008.

Bulkeley, K. Reflections on the dream traditions of Islam. *Sleep and Hypnosis*. 2002; 4:4–14.

Cohen, S., N. Kozlovsky, M. A. Matar, et al. Post-exposure sleep deprivation facilitates correctly timed interactions between glucocorticoid and adrenergic systems, which attenuate traumatic stress responses. *Neuropsychopharmacology*. 2012; 37 (11):2388–404.

Coutts, R. Dreams as modifiers and tests of mental schemas: An emotional selection hypothesis. *Psychological Reports*. 2008; 102 (2):561–74.

Crick, F., and G. Mitchison. The function of dream sleep. *Nature*. 1983; 304 (5922):111–14.

Dyer, W. How do you sleep? *DrWayneDyer.com* (blog). http://www.drwaynedyer.com/blog/how-do-you-sleep/.

Fausbøll, V., and D. Andersen. *The Jataka: Together with Its Commentary, Being Tales of the Anterior Births of Gotama Buddha*. Vol. 6. (London: Trübner & Co., 1896).

Firewolf, D. The history of dreaming—from ancient Egypt to modern day. *Realmagick.com* (blog), 2011.

Freud, S. *The Interpretation of Dreams*. Translated by James Strachey. New York: Basic Books, 2010 (1900).

Gallop, D. *Aristotle on Sleep and Dreams*. Warminster, UK: Aris & Phillips, 1996.

Gillis, L. And now a word from ancient Egypt. . . . *Dreaminglucid.com* (blog), 2009.

Hartmann, E. The underlying emotion and the dream: Relating dream imagery to the dreamer's underlying emotion can help elucidate the nature of dreaming. *International Review of Neurobiology*. 2010; 92:197–214.

Heraclitus. *Fragments: A Text and Translation with a Commentary*. Translated by T. M. Robinson. Toronto: University of Toronto Press, 1987.

Hobson, J. A., and R. W. McCarley. The brain as a dream state generator: An activation-synthesis hypothesis of the dream process. *American Journal of Psychiatry*. 1977; 134 (12):1335–48.

Newitz, A., and J. Bennington-Castro. 10 theories that explain why we dream. *Gizmodo.com* (blog), 2013. http://io9.gizmodo.com/10-theories-that-explain-why-we-dream-897195110.

Ong, R. K. *The Interpretation of Dreams in Ancient China* (master of arts thesis). Vancouver, Canada: University of British Columbia; 1981.

Plato. Crito. In E. Hamilton and H. Cairns, eds. *Plato: Collected Dialogues*. Princeton, NJ: Princeton University Press, 1961.

Plato. *The Republic*. In B. Jowett, ed. *The Dialogues of Plato*. Vol. 2. Fourth edition. Oxford: Clarendon Press, 1953, 1–499.

Pollak, C., M. J. Thorpy, and J. Yager. *The Encyclopedia of Sleep and Sleep Disorders*. Third edition. New York: Facts on File, 2009.

Revonsuo, A. The reinterpretation of dreams: An evolutionary hypothesis of the function of dreaming. *The Behavioral and Brain Sciences*. 2000; 23 (6):877–901.

Schredl, M. Characteristics and contents of dreams. *International Review of Neurobiology*. 2010; 92:135–54.

Tolle, E. *The Power of Now: A Guide to Spiritual Enlightenment*. Vancouver, BC: Namaste Publishing, 1999.

Wamsley, E. J., and R. Stickgold. Dreaming and offline memory processing. *Current Biology*. 2010; 20 (23):R1010–13.

Wamsley, E. J., M. Tucker, J. D. Payne, et al. Dreaming of a learning task is associated with enhanced sleep-dependent memory consolidation. *Current Biology*. 2010; 20 (9):850–55.

Young, S. Buddhist dream experience. In K. Bulkeley, ed. *Dreams: A Reader on Religious, Cultural and Psychological Dimensions of Dreaming*. New York: Palgrave Macmillan, 2001.

Zhang, J. Continual-activation theory of dreaming. *Dynamical Psychology*. 2005.

Conclusion

Barone, D. A., and A. C. Krieger. The function of sleep. *AIMS Neuroscience*. 2015; 2 (2): 71–90.

ADDITIONAL RESOURCES

The following organizations and websites contain information that is useful for both patients and their doctors. Among other things, they provide updates on research studies.

American Sleep Apnea Foundation; https://www.sleepapnea.org
Hypersomnia Foundation; http://www.hypersomniafoundation.org/
National Heart, Lung, and Blood Institute (NHLBI); http://www.nhlbi.nih.gov
National Organization for Rare Disorders (NORD); http://www.rarediseases.org
National Sleep Foundation; https://sleepfoundation.org/
Restless Legs Syndrome Foundation; http://www.rls.org/
Sleep Education: A Sleep Health Information Resource by the American Academy of Sleep Medicine; http://www.sleepeducation.org

In addition, these free resources provide time zone data that are helpful when you travel:

http://www.jetlagrooster.com
http://www.timeanddate.com

While we have not cited the following books and medical journals specifically, they provide a wealth of useful background information.

Arzt, M., T. Young, L. Finn, et al. Association of sleep-disordered breathing and the occurrence of stroke. *American Journal of Respiratory and Critical Care Medicine*. 2005; 172 (11):1447–51.
Attal, P., and P. Chanson. Endocrine aspects of obstructive sleep apnea. *Journal of clinical endocrinology and metabolism*. 2010; 95 (2):483–95.
Barone, D. A., and A. C. Krieger. Stroke and obstructive sleep apnea: A review. *Current Atherosclerosis Reports*. 2013; 15 (7):334.
Benito-Leon, J., F. Bermejo-Pareja, S. Vega, and E. D. Louis. Total daily sleep duration and the risk of dementia: A prospective population-based study. *European Journal of Neurology*. 2009; 16 (9): 990–97.
Blackwell, T., K. Yaffe, S. Ancoli-Israel, et al. Poor sleep is associated with impaired cognitive function in older women: The study of osteoporotic fractures. *Journals of Gerontology: Series A, Biological Sciences and Medical Sciences*. 2006; 61 (4): 405–10.
Brondel, L., M. A. Romer, P. M. Nogues, et al. Acute partial sleep deprivation increases food intake in healthy men. *American Journal of Clinical Nutrition*. 2010; 91 (6):1550–59.
Bulpitt, C. J., K. Shaw, P. Clifton, et al. The symptoms of patients treated for Parkinson's disease. *Clinical Neuropharmacology*. 1985; 8 (2):175–83.
Chokroverty, S. Diagnosis and treatment of sleep disorders caused by co-morbid disease. *Neurology*. 2000; 54 (5) suppl. 1:S8-15.

Das, A. M., and M. Khan. Obstructive sleep apnea and stroke. *Expert review of cardiovascular therapy.* 2012; 10 (4):525–35.

Dement, W. C. *Some Must Watch While Some Must Sleep.* New York: Books on Tape, Inc., 1974.

Dement, W. C. *The Promise of Sleep.* New York, NY: Dell Publishing, 1999.

Dement, W. C. *The Stanford Sleep Book.* Fifth edition. N.P.: Author, 2006.

Durmer, J. S. and D. F. Dinges. Neurocognitive consequences of sleep deprivation. *Seminars in Neurology.* 2005; 25 (1):117–29.

Fiorentini, A., J. Ora, and L. Tubani. Autonomic system modification in Zen practitioners. *Indian Journal of Medical Sciences.* 2013; 67 (7–8):161–67.

Gangwisch, J. E., S. B. Heymsfield, B. Boden-Albala, et al. Short sleep duration as a risk factor for hypertension: Analyses of the first National Health and Nutrition Examination Survey. *Hypertension.* 2006; 47 (5):833–39.

Havekes, R., C. G. Vecsey, and T. Abel. The impact of sleep deprivation on neuronal and glial signaling pathways important for memory and synaptic plasticity. *Cellular Signalling.* 2012; 24 (6):1251–60.

Helbig, A. K., D. Stöckl, M. Heier, et al. Symptoms of insomnia and sleep duration and their association with incident strokes: Findings from the population-based MONICA/KORA Augsburg Cohort Study. *PLoS.* 2015; 10 (7):e0134480.

Holowchak, M. A. Interpreting dreams for corrective regimen: Diagnostic dreams in Greco-Roman medicine. *Journal of the History of Medicine and Allied Sciences.* 2001; 56 (4):382–99.

Hossain, J. L., and C. M. Shapiro. The prevalence, cost implications, and management of sleep disorders: An overview. *Sleep and Breathing.* 2002; 6 (2):85–102.

Hsu, C. Y., Y. T. Chen, M. H. Chen, et al. The association between insomnia and increased future cardiovascular events: A nationwide population-based study. *Psychosomatic Medicine.* 2015; 77 (7):743–51.

Hudgel, D. W. Mechanisms of obstructive sleep apnea. *Chest.* 1992; 101 (2):541–49.

Jennum, P., and R. Jensen. Sleep and headache. *Sleep Medicine Reviews.* 2002; 6 (6):471–79.

Kan, L. B. Introduction to Chinese medical literature. *Bulletin of the Medical Library Association.* 1965; 53:60–70.

Katz, D. A., and C. A. McHorney. Clinical correlates of insomnia in patients with chronic illness. *Archives of Internal Medicine.* 1985; 158 (10):1099–107.

Kothare, S. V., and A. Ivanenko. Introduction. In S. V. Kothare and A. Ivanenko, eds. *Parasomnias.* New York: Springer Science+Business Media, 2013.

Kryger, M. H., ed. *Atlas of Clinical Sleep Medicine.* Philadelphia: Saunders, 2010.

Kryger, M. H., and T. Roth, eds. *Principles and Practice of Sleep Medicine.* Sixth edition. Philadelphia: Elsevier, 2017.

Kufoy, E., J. A. Palma, J. Lopez, et al. Changes in the heart rate variability in patients with obstructive sleep apnea and its response to acute CPAP treatment. *PLoS.* 2012; 7 (3): e33769.

Kuppermann, M. Sleep problems and their correlates in a working population. *Journal of General Internal Medicine.* 1995; 10 (1):25–32.

Laugsand, L. E., L. J. Vatten, C. Platou, and I. Janszky. Insomnia and the risk of acute myocardial infarction: A population study. *Circulation.* 2011; 124 (19):2073–81.

López-Muñoz, F., J. D. Molina, G. Rubio, and C. Alamo. An historical view of the pineal gland and mental disorders. *Journal of Clinical Neuroscience.* 2011; 8:1028–37.

Malow, B. A. The interaction between sleep and epilepsy. *Epilepsia.* 2007; 48, suppl 9: 36–38.

Manenschijn, L., R. G. van Kruysbergen, F. H. deJong, et al. Shift work at young age is associated with elevated long-term cortisol levels and body mass index. *Journal of Clinical Endocrinology and Metabolism.* 2011; 96 (11):e1862-5.

Mansfield, R., S. Goddard, and H. Moldofsky. "When the external fire departs": Sleep theories of Plato and Aristotle and their relevance to modern sleep research. *University of Toronto Medical Journal.* 2003; 81 (1).

Moldofsky, H. Sleep and pain. *Sleep Medicine Reviews.* 2001; 5 (5):385–96.

Morin, C. M., D. Gibson, and J. Wade. Self-reported sleep and mood disturbance in chronic pain patients. *Clinical Journal of Pain*. 1998; 14 (4):311–14.

Muñoz, R., J. Durán-Cantolla, E. Martinez-Vila, et al. Central sleep apnea is associated with increased risk of ischemic stroke in the elderly. *Acta Neurologica Scandinavica*. 2012; 126 (3):183–88.

Nieto, F. J., T. B. Young, B. K. Lind, et al. Association of sleep-disordered breathing, sleep apnea, and hypertension in a large community-based study. Sleep Heart Health Study. *Journal of the American Medical Association*. 2000; 283 (14):1829–36.

Pagel, J. F. What physicians need to know about dreams and dreaming. *Current Opinion in Pulmonary Medicine*. 2012; 18 (6):574–79.

Palagini, L., and N. Rosenlicht. Sleep, dreaming, and mental health: A review of historical and neurobiological perspectives. *Sleep Medicine Reviews*. 2011; 15 (3):179–86.

Palma, J. A., E. Urrestarazu, and J. Iriarte. Sleep loss as risk factor for neurologic disorders: A review. *Sleep Medicine*. 2013; 14 (3):229–36.

Patil, S. P., H. Schneider, A. R. Schwartz, and P. L. Smith. Adult obstructive sleep apnea: Pathophysiology and diagnosis. *Chest*. 2007; 132 (1):325–37.

Pilowsky, I., I. Crettenden, and M. Townley. Sleep disturbance in pain clinic patients. *Pain*. 1985; 23 (1):27–33.

Rains, J. C., J. S. Poceta, and D. B. Penzien. Sleep and headaches. *Current Neurology and Neuroscience Reports*. 2008; 8 (2):167–75.

Rechtschaffen, A. Current perspectives on the function of sleep. *Perspectives in Biology and Medicine*. 1998; 41 (3):359–90.

Roehrs, T., M. Hyde, B. Blaisdell, et al. Sleep loss and REM sleep loss are hyperalgesic. *Sleep*. 2006; 29 (2):145–51.

Shahar, E., C. W. Whitney, S. Redline, et al. Sleep-disordered breathing and cardiovascular disease: Cross-sectional results of the Sleep Heart Health Study. *American Journal of Respiratory and Critical Care Medicine*. 2001; 163 (1):19–25.

Smith, M. T., R. R. Edwards, U. D. McCann, and J. A. Haythornthwaite. The effects of sleep deprivation on pain inhibition and spontaneous pain in women. *Sleep*. 2007; 30 (4): 494–505.

Sofi, F., F. Cesari, A. Casini, et al. Insomnia and risk of cardiovascular disease: A meta-analysis. *European Journal of Preventive Cardiology*. 2014; 21 (1):57–64.

Somers, V. K., M. E. Dyken, M. P. Clary, and F. M. Abboud. Sympathetic neural mechanisms in obstructive sleep apnea. *Journal of Clinical Investigations*. 1995; 96 (4):1897–904.

Spiegel, K., K. Knutson, R. Leproult, et al. Sleep loss: A novel risk factor for insulin resistance and Type 2 diabetes. *Journal of Applied Physiology*. 2005; 99 (5):2008–19.

Spiegel, K., E. Tasali, R. Leproult, and E. Van Cauter. Effects of poor and short sleep on glucose metabolism and obesity risk. *Nature Reviews: Endocrinology*. 2009; 5 (5):253–61.

Spira, A. P., T. Blackweel, K. L. Stone, et al. Sleep-disordered breathing and cognition in older women. *Journal of the American Geriatric Society*. 2008; 56 (1):45–50.

Tranah, G. J., T. Blackweel, K. L. Stone, et al. Circadian activity rhythms and risk of incident dementia and mild cognitive impairment in older women. *Annals of Neurology*. 2011; 70 (5):722–32.

Tworoger, S. S., S. Lee, E. S. Schernhammer, and F. Grodstein. The association of self-reported sleep duration, difficulty sleeping, and snoring with cognitive function in older women. *Alzheimer Disease and Associated Disorders*. 2006; 20 (1):41–48.

Van Dongen, H., G. Maislin, J. M. Mullington, and D. F. Dinges. The cumulative cost of additional wakefulness: Dose-response effects on neurobehavioral functions and sleep physiology from chronic sleep restriction and total sleep deprivation. *Sleep*. 2003; 26 (2):117–26.

Vyas, M. V., A. X. Garg, A. Vlansavichus, et al. Shift work and vascular events: Systematic review and meta-analysis. *British Medical Journal*. 2012; 345:e4800.

Walker, M. P. Cognitive consequences of sleep and sleep loss. *Sleep Medicine*. 2008; 9, suppl 1: S29-34.

Walters, A. S., and D. B. Rye. Review of the relationship of restless legs syndrome and periodic limb movements in sleep to hypertension, heart disease, and stroke. *Sleep*. 32 (5): 589–97.

Willoughby, B. B., J. R. Lindahl, B. R. Cahn, et al. Awakening is not a metaphor: The effects of Buddhist meditation practices on basic wakefulness. *Annals of the New York Academy of Sciences*. 2014; 1307:64–81.

Wilson, K. G., M. Y. Eriksson, J. L. D'Eon, et al. Major depression and insomnia in chronic pain. *Clinical Journal of Pain*. 2002; 18 (2):77–83.

Yaggi, H. K., J. Concato, W. N. Kernan, et al. Obstructive sleep apnea as a risk factor for stroke and death. *New England Journal of Medicine*. 2005; 353 (19):2034–41.

Zammit, G. K., J. Weiner, N. Damato, et al. Quality of life in people with insomnia. *Sleep*. 1999; 22, suppl 2:S379–85.

INDEX

health: blood pressure, 5; consequences
    of, 17–18, 41; of heart, 2–3; impact on,
    139–140. *See also* mental problems;
    weight
heart, 2–3
Hinduism, 136
Hippocrates, 29
history: in Ancient China, 2–3; in Ancient
    Greece, 1; in Bible, 1; interest
    throughout, 3; in Islam, 1–2; of
    narcolepsy, 101; in Old Testament, 2;
    pineal gland in, 12; of Valerian, 48–49
hormones, 48
humans: biology of, 30; differences in,
    12–13; dissection of, 12; ideal hours
    for, 33–34; risk for, 15
hygiene, 113–114, 161; as solution, 45;
    value of, 2, 30
hypervigilance, 30
hypnagogic/hypnopompic hallucinations,
    24, 158
Hypnos, 1
hypnotic, 158
hypocretin, 158
hypoglossal nerve, 158
hypoglossal nerve stimulation, 67, 158
hypothalamus, 106–107, 158
hypoventilation, 77, 79, 158
hypoxemia, 76–77, 79, 158

I Can See Clearly Now (Dyer), 137
ICSD-3. *See The International
    Classification of Sleep Disorders—
    Third Edition*
idiopathic hypersomnia, 26, 109–110, 159.
    See also narcolepsy
idiopathic insomnia, 36
The Iliad (Homer), 1
insomnia: age of, 36; anxiety and, 44;
    definition of, 29; depression and, 44;
    development of, 34; experience of, 2;
    morale of, 36; solutions for, 7; torment
    of, 32; variations of, 38. *See also* acute
    insomnia; chronic insomnia
insurance, 3, 26
internal clock, 7. *See also* circadian
    rhythm
*The International Classification of Sleep
    Disorders—Third Edition* (ICSD-3),

98
The Interpretation of Dreams (Freud),
    130
Islam, 1–2

jet lag, 120, 159; treatment for, 121–122,
    123
John (doctor), 118–119
John (patient), 82–84
Jordan (patient), 34–36
journaling, 19, 41–42, 125

Linda (patient), 102–103
Lisa (patient), 71–73
"long sleeper", 13
lucid dreaming, 134
Lunesta. *See* eszopiclone
lymphatic system, 157–158

MAD. *See* mandibular advancement de-
    vice
magnesium, 50, 85
Mallampati score, 21
mandibular advancement device (MAD),
    62, 63, 159; adjustments for, 63; risks
    of, 64
Mark (patient), 71–73
Marlene (patient), 40–41
medical costs. *See* insurance
medications. *See* prescription medication;
    remedies; stimulant medications
meditation: of Buddhist monks, 13;
    instructions for, 9–10; as solution, 31,
    32, 63; variations of, 9. *See also*
    mindfulness meditation
melatonin, 42, 43, 48, 117, 159; as
    antioxidant, 48; as hormone, 48; as
    natural remedy, 48; safety of, 48; use
    of, 48
mental problems, 23
methadone, 83, 85–86
Michael (patient), 62–64
mindfulness meditation, 10; as solution, 9,
    39
mothers: after pregnancy, 31; MSLT. *See*
    multiple sleep latency test
Muhammad, 1–2
multiple sleep latency test (MSLT), 26,
    107, 159

ABOUT THE AUTHORS

Daniel A. Barone, MD, is currently an assistant professor of neurology at Weill Cornell Medical College. He primarily sees patients at the Weill Cornell Medical College Center for Sleep Medicine, where he specializes in the evaluation and management of patients with all forms of sleep disorders, including sleep apnea, restless legs syndrome, insomnia, and narcolepsy. He is certified by the American Board of Psychiatry and Neurology in both Neurology and Sleep Medicine, and is a member of the American Academy of Neurology and a fellow of the American Academy of Sleep Medicine. Dr. Barone is frequently featured in the media; he has appeared on various television programs, including *CBS Nightly News* regarding the Centers for Disease Control and Prevention's report that single moms have reduced sleep compared to those in two-parent households, as well as Discovery Channel's popular *Deadliest Catch: The Bait* as an expert in sleep disorders. He has been quoted in articles in *Reader's Digest, Prevention, New York Daily News, Allure, Healthline, Time*, and *Self*. Dr. Barone also is involved in sleep research and has published numerous peer-reviewed articles.

Lawrence A. Armour left Time Inc. in August 2015 and has since built a freelance writing and editing business focused on magazines, newspapers, corporations, and individual authors. Armour spent sixteen years in various positions at Time Inc. Prior to that, he worked in communications at IBM, American Express, and Dow Jones. A graduate of Dartmouth College and an MBA graduate of Northwestern University, he began his career at *Barron's*, first as a reporter and then as an associate editor and columnist. Armour's first book, *Profits on Wall Street*, was followed by three others: *Investing for Profit, How to Survive a Bear Market*, and *Managing to Succeed*. Other books include *The Young Millionaires; How to Make Your Money Make Money*, written with Arthur Levitt Jr.; and *The RealAge Workout*, written with Dr. Michael F. Roizen and Tracy Hafen.